Geriatric Gastroenterology

WILLIAM A. SODEMAN, JR., M.D.

Associate Dean for Academic Affairs
Louisiana State University Medical Center
School of Medicine in Shreveport
Shreveport, Louisiana

THOMAS A. SALADIN, M.D.

Associate Medical Director
Director, Department of Medicine
Good Samaritan Hospital
Cincinnati, Ohio

WILLIAM P. BOYD, JR., M.D.

Clinical Associate Professor of Medicine
Department of Internal Medicine
University of South Florida
Tampa, Florida

1989

W.B. SAUNDERS COMPANY
Harcourt Brace Jovanovich, Inc.
Philadelphia, San Diego, London, Toronto, Montreal, Sydney, Tokyo

W. B. SAUNDERS COMPANY
Harcourt Brace Jovanovich, Inc.

The Curtis Center
Independence Square West
Philadelphia, PA 19106

Library of Congress Cataloging-in-Publication Data

Sodeman, William A. (William Anthony). 1936–   .

Geriatric gastroenterology/William A. Sodeman, Jr.,
William P. Boyd, Jr., Thomas A. Saladin.

p. cm.

1. Geriatric gastroenterology.   2. Gastrointestinal system—
Diseases—Age factors.   I. Boyd, William P.
II. Saladin, Thomas A., 1933–   .   III. Title.
[DNLM: 1. Gastrointestinal Diseases—in old age. WI 100
S679g]

RC802.4.A34S63 1989   618.97′633—dc19   88–39827

DNLM/DLC

ISBN 0–7216–2799–4

Acquisition Editor: John Dyson
Designer: Joan Sinclair
Production Manager: Frank Polizzano
Manuscript Editor: Keryn Lane
Indexer: Julie Palmeter

Geriatric Gastroenterology   ISBN   0–7216–2799–4

Printed in the United States of America.

Last digit is the print number: 9   8   7   6   5   4   3   2   1

Preface

This short book was written with the needs of the primary care physician in mind. There are excellent encyclopedic texts on geriatrics, gastroenterology, and geriatric gastroenterology. The literature is also replete with highly specific papers on various gastrointestinal and hepatic problems in the elderly. What has been missing is a brief presentation that can serve as an introduction to the topic of digestive tract problems in the elderly and remain a handy guide in the management of these patients. There is no intent to substitute for either the "encyclopedias" or the papers, rather to simplify the introduction to them.

Brevity implies that we have selected to include some problems and to defer discussion of others. For the most part the inclusions are common problems and deferrals were limited to rare and unusual problems. The selection of material to be presented has focused on diagnosis and management. We have eschewed basic and research issues unless they carry immediate clinical relevance. In addition, where the literature remains confusing and issues are unresolved, we have sought to call attention to this to prevent the physician from being gulled by a reasonable sounding explanation in the absence of confirmatory data.

The authors acknowledge the support of their families and the help of their secretaries in the preparation of the manuscript. We also acknowledge our elderly patients for their inspiration and contribution to the development of this volume.

WILLIAM A. SODEMAN, JR., M.D.

THOMAS A. SALADIN, M.D.

WILLIAM P. BOYD, JR., M.D.

Contents

Chapter 1

THE ESOPHAGUS

Thomas A. Saladin

A discussion of esophageal disease in the elderly often focuses on carcinoma, but motility disorders and even congenital abnormalities may first make their appearance in older patients (Pelemans & Vantrappen, 1985). This chapter, therefore, includes a discussion of SIDES (symptomatic, idiopathic, diffuse, esophageal spasm) and achalasia but primarily highlights in the diseases described, features that are of special importance, in the geriatric population.

Ordinarily I like to classify dysphagia, the principal symptom of esophageal disease, using normal esophageal physiology as the foundation of division. Thus, *transfer* is applied to the early, partially voluntary phase of the swallow when food is propelled by the tongue to the upper esophagus. *Transport* is defined as the movement of the bolus along the esophagus from the cricopharyngeus to the lower esophageal sphincter (LES); and *entrance* refers to the passage of material from the esophagus to the stomach. This chapter is roughly divided according to this classification since motility abnormalities cause transfer and transport dysphagia, and structural abnormalities cause entrance dysphagia. Some diseases cause all three. The clinical importance of the classification is to help one decide which diseases are most likely to be responsible for certain symptoms. Examples will be discussed in appropriate parts of the chapter. Treatment will be outlined, but some of the more technical considerations are left for the gastroenterologist or surgeon.

1

MOTILITY DISORDERS

Motility disorders are fairly common in the aged, particularly if one includes those that are asymptomatic or are caused by a more important illness such as diabetes mellitus or Parkinson's disease. They can be investigated by barium esophagram, cineradiography, endoscopy, or manometrics—each diagnostic tool has its place. One should suspect disordered motility as the cause of the patient's problem when the complaint is aspiration, nasal regurgitation of the bolus which is worse with liquids than solids (transfer dysphagia), or dysphagia for liquids and solids with some relief afforded when a Valsalva maneuver is done or when the arms are held over the head (transport dysphagia).

Mensuration

Devices for measuring these motor phenomena have been in common use for more than 35 years (Kramer & Ingelfinger, 1949) and have been particularly popular since the publication of the work of Code and colleagues (1958) concerning esophageal motility. Most of the devices are constructed so that the propagation of the peristaltic wave down the esophagus can be measured at three points, each placed 5 cm aborally from its predecessor. This may be accomplished by transducers fixed on a tube that is swallowed or by construction of a triple lumen tube with occlusion of each lumen distal to its side port, which is located 5 cm distal to the side port in the previous lumen. Connected to a transducer and filled with water, each lumen receives pressure transmitted to its portal during activity of the esophagus. The corresponding transducer changes the signal to an electrical impulse that can be measured and recorded on paper for permanent storage. More accurate and attractive recordings can be made if the whole system is filled with water perfused by a high pressure system (Arndorfer, et al., 1977). This is particularly true of measurements of LES pressure and activity. Such devices work less well in the upper sphincter because of coughing caused by the water load in the hypopharynx.

The method is especially well suited to measuring and recording the activities of the body of the esophagus. It also gives manometric information about the upper sphincter. Because the upper esophageal musculature is striated, its contractions are very fast; cine-esophagography with its picture rate of 30 to 60 frames per second is better suited to the task of documenting most events in this area including the identification of aspiration caused by dysfunction of the cricopharyngeal muscles.

Classification

Transfer Dysphagia

In geriatric practice, one sometimes encounters patients who complain of dysphagia in an area referred to as the "Adam's apple." While difficulty swallowing perceived in that location can be referred from the lower esophagus, one should think of causes of a transfer abnormality as well. These include *neurological diseases* such as brainstem infarcts, parkinsonism, Guillain-Barré syndrome, amyotrophic lateral sclerosis, multiple sclerosis, and cervical trauma; *muscular diseases* such as dermatomyositis, myasthenia gravis, and myotonia dystrophica; and *metabolic diseases,* particularly diabetes mellitus and hypo- and hyperthyroidism (Fischer, et al., 1965).

Neurological Diseases

Neurological disorders of the esophagus have in common interference with the voluntary and reflux control of the striated muscles supplied by cranial nerves V, IX, X, and XII, for these are the ones used to transfer food and drink from the mouth to the hypopharynx. In the case of Parkinson's disease, dysphagia is caused by slowness and incoordination of the muscles rather than by partial or complete paralysis.

Muscular Diseases

Although muscular diseases affect striated muscle, smooth muscle can also be abnormal as in dermatomyositis which is related to scleroderma. Myotonia dystrophica, like dermatomyositis, also affects smooth muscle of the esophagus. The resulting disorder is more complex in these two cases. Hyper- and hypothyroidism are also examples of disorders that cause complex abnormalities of both smooth and striated muscle function, with or without symptoms, related to transfer, transport, or both. Usually each of these maladies is readily diagnosed, but one must be aware of the relationship of the disease to dysphagia and consider it in the differential diagnosis. Physical findings that help confirm the condition can then be sought and appropriate tests made to complete the diagnosis.

Treatment. Treatment of some neurological disorders is specific. In contrast, brainstem infarcts and cervical trauma require physical therapy until maximum achievable control is attained. Sometimes this can be augmented by a cricopharyngeal myotomy as described below. The dysphagia associated with Parkinson's disease may respond to treatment with L-dopa (Cotzias, et al., 1969) or with other, standard medicines used for the disease. Amyotrophic lateral sclerosis and multiple sclerosis are usually unyielding.

The muscle diseases, on the other hand, may respond in a gratifying way—dermatomyositis to corticosteroids, myasthenia to cholinesterase inhibitors, and myotonia to quinine. Improvement due to treatment of thyroid diseases is more predictable and complete.

Primary Dysfunction of the Cricopharyngeus

Cricopharyngeal dysfunction occurs at all ages but seems especially prone to attack the elderly in whom it can be associated with Zenker's diverticulum, a saccular outpouching of the pharyngeal wall through the fibers of the cricopharyngeus, often on the right side. Review of the anatomy of the pharynx reminds one that there are some spaces between the middle and inferior constrictors which subject the area to the possibility of herniation. If during swallowing the cricopharyngeus does not relax in a timely way, the pressure in the hypopharynx may reach a high level. Offered as an explanation for formation of Zenker's diverticulum, this hypothesis has not been proven to everyone's satisfaction (van Overbeck, 1977).

Manometric investigation of these patients may show that the upper esophageal sphincter fails to relax completely and/or in synchrony with the other muscles of deglutition. It may also be normal! Cine-esophagography is probably a better diagnostic tool, but any and all methods of investigation sometimes fail to make the diagnosis. The patient may then erroneously be labeled "neurotic," a sufferer from globus hystericus. Since treatment of malfunction of the cricopharyngeus is reasonably effective, one would like to avoid this error.

Treatment. Treatment of cricopharyngeal dysfunction may be as simple as reassurance when aspiration and weight loss are absent and symptoms are minor. Dilatation with a mercury-filled bougie also works, but stubborn symptoms associated with weight loss and aspiration require cricopharyngeal sphincterotomy. This operation can be performed through a neck incision; it is ordinarily safe and easily done when one observes the precaution of assuring that serious gastroesophageal reflux is absent. In addition to its use in the treatment of the patients under discussion, cricopharyngeal section has met with some success for those suffering from stroke, Parkinson's disease, and other neurological ailments, particularly when sensation is intact.

Other Considerations. In order to avoid error, one must consider the structural lesions that can mimic cricopharyngeal dysfunction, either idiopathic or secondary to one of the diseases mentioned above. These disorders include muscle damage; nerve damage; scars due to previous surgical manipulation in the neck; webs; Plummer-Vinson syndrome; Zenker's diverticulum; carcinoma of the larynx, hypopharynx, or upper esophagus; and extrinsic lesions that compress the area, e.g., abscess, thyromegaly, cervical lymphadenopathy, and hyperostosis of the cervical spine.

If one avoids these pitfalls and faithfully observes the indications for treatment, results of cricopharyngeal section will be good in idiopathic malfunction of the upper sphincter and the related Zenker's diverticulum, excellent in the rare oculopharyngeal dystrophy, variably good in central or peripheral nervous system disease when sensation is intact, and variable in dysfunction due to surgical disease depending on the kind of damage. Complications include sudden death (due to aspiration?); bleeding, which has been rare and not troublesome; perforation; recurrent laryngeal nerve palsy; mediastinitis; aerophagia; and esophageal breathing, which causes unpleasant and embarrassing belching but is not dangerous. There have been no reports of inadequate section.

Transport Dysphagia

When transport dysphagia is present, one must consider a different but overlapping group of diseases, the most important of which are symptomatic, idiopathic, diffuse, esophageal spasm (SIDES) and achalasia. Both are considered diseases of younger persons (20 to 40 years of age), but they can occur in the elderly in whom they evoke fear of cancer. Such fears are well founded as dicussed below.

SIDES (Symptomatic, Idiopathic, Diffuse, Esophageal Spasm)

SIDES is common or rare depending upon the criteria used to diagnose it. If one demands episodes of severe, angina-like chest pain and dysphagia accompanied by markedly elevated pressures in the body of the esophagus during passage of a nonperistaltic wave, the syndrome will be rare. If pressures higher than 200 mm Hg are not required, but merely nonperistaltic waves with or without chest pain, the disease will be more common. No matter how confusing, the disease does exist and must be considered in the differential diagnosis of dysphagia and chest pain (Clause, et al., 1983), particularly when a transport abnormality is suggested by the clinical history.

Manometric Criteria. Cattau and Castell (1982) have required the following criteria in 30 per cent or more of contractions measured manometrically: three or more contractions in response to a swallow, simultaneous waves, and contractions lasting longer than 7 seconds. Associated findings comprise hypertension of the LES, incomplete relaxation of the LES during a swallow, and high amplitude (>200 mm Hg) contractions in the body of the esophagus.

Differential Diagnosis. Once manometric investigation has determined the presence of SIDES, the physician must discover whether any of the causes of this abnormality are present. The minimum requirement is a search for esophagitis because it can be treated effectively and has management requirements different from SIDES, which by definition is idiopathic. Scleroderma (Saladin, et al., 1966) and other connective tissue diseases also cause nonperistaltic contractions in the body of the esophagus in response to swallowing. In these conditions and in thyrotoxicosis, diabetes (Mandelstane & Lieber, 1967), Parkinson's disease, and other neurological diseases, the pressure of the waves in the body of the esophagus is usually low. Clause and Lustman (1983) demonstrated similar abnormalities in a group of psychiatric patients, only 25 per cent of whom had normal manometry of the esophagus. Most of these disorders are worth knowing about when one is caring for a patient; therefore, they should be considered when a motility disturbance is diagnosed.

Of course, when chest pain is the most significant manifestation of SIDES, differentiation from angina pectoris is critical and difficult. Both syndromes may give identical pain which can be relieved by nitroglycerine and which may be accompanied by coronary artery disease. In the elderly the differentiation is even more important and confusing, especially since the pain of SIDES has occasionally been associated with exercise (Richter, et al., 1985). The problem has resulted in attempts to develop provocative tests for borderline cases (Benjamin, et al., 1983). It is better to miss the diagnosis of SIDES than that of coronary artery disease because the former has a good prognosis; but one would be disgruntled to find that a coronary artery bypass graft failed to relieve the symptoms of the patient only to discover that SIDES was the cause of the chest pain.

Treatment. Having cleared all of these hurdles, the physician may now wonder whether effective treatment can be offered to the patient with SIDES. Removal of precipitating stimuli should be prescribed first. These stimuli may be emotional or physical. Pleasantness at meals is not only polite, but it is also therapeutic; it should not be overlooked. If reflux is a trigger, antacids or other measures to reduce acid should be tried. Proscription of carbonated, hot, or cold beverages may be effective. Other ingested stimulants should be searched for and removed—with the physician always being careful to avoid blanket condemnation of foods and beverages that do not, in that particular patient, cause trouble.

Failure of these simple, cost-free measures should signal the need for a trial of short- or long-acting nitrates, followed by calcium channel blocking agents (Traube, et al., 1984). Diltiazem is recommended because of the paucity of side effects (Richter, et al., 1984), but both classes of drugs relax smooth muscle and do not differentiate between esophageal and coronary artery musculature. Their effectiveness in SIDES is not proved, but anecdotal information suggests that they be used for now.

For the patient whose disease resists all these treatments, one can recommend mercury bougienage with a large-sized instrument (60F). Since it passes with ease and does not tear anything, one wonders why it is effective in some patients. Once again, acceptable studies have not proven the worth of the bougie, so an open mind is required.

When all else fails, an esophageal myotomy, similar to that used for the treatment of achalasia, is indicated. The incision of the esophageal muscle is carried almost to the aortic arch. Results are usually good, but reflux esophagitis may occur (due to poor acid clearing?); therefore, when the lower esophageal sphincter pressure (LESP) is low, some surgeons recommend an anti-reflux procedure as well (Sleisinger, 1983). Proof for the validity of this recommendation is incomplete. Because of the uncertainty about treatment considerations, physicians will want a high degree of certainty about the diagnosis in their patients. Therefore, before undertaking surgical treatments, I recommend a strict interpretation of the manometric records and a thorough consideration of, if not testing for, other diagnostic possibilities, particularly angina, esophagitis, or other treatable conditions.

Achalasia

Also unusual in this age group, achalasia is better defined than SIDES both clinically and manometrically. It is more frequently associated with radiographic changes (Kraft, et al., 1973) which consist of dilatation of the body of the esophagus, often with an air-fluid level, and narrowing (parrot beak) of the LES (Fig. 1–1). This narrow area is easily passed by a bougie or endoscope in contrast to narrowing caused by peptic strictures or cancer.

Manometric Criteria. Manometric criteria for the diagnosis of achalasia, include absence of peristalsis in the body of the esophagus, low amplitude or absent waves in the body of the esophagus, and high-pressure LES that does not relax during swallowing. An esophagus affected by achalasia contracts forcefully in response to cholinergic stimulation by drugs such as Mecholyl or Urecholine. This behavior is thought to be a manifestation of Cannon's law of denervation which states that organs supplied by the autonomic nervous system become supersensitive to the chemical mediator of their nervous supply.

Pharmacological tests are no longer performed routinely; Mecholyl is now not available, and the test was uncomfortable. In addition, the exact manometric and clinical features just described can be caused by carcinoma of the cardia, presumably because of invasion of Auerbach's plexus by the neoplasm. The clinical caveat that results from this fact

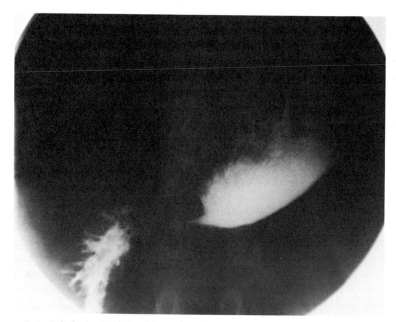

Figure 1–1. Achalasia. Note in this reversed image the narrow segment in the area of the lower esophageal sphincter. It never opens, but a dilator will pass through it without difficulty. Carcinoma of the cardia may produce an identical radiograph. Compare this dilated esophagus with the one of scleroderma in Figure 1–2.

is to suspect carcinoma of the cardia in older patients who present themselves with "achalasia." Upper gastrointestinal panendoscopy is required in such patients, and special efforts should be made to view the cardia by means of the retroflex maneuver. Nevertheless, achalasia is possible in the elderly; I have seen it become manifest in the ninth decade.

Pathophysiology. The reason for the motor abnormalities seen in achalasia is not entirely known. Surely, the absence of Auerbach's plexus in the muscularis of the esophagus explains the lack of effective, peristaltic, muscular contraction in the body of the organ. The same abnormality is acquired in Chagas' disease, which produces identical clinical and manometric findings. The changes in the function of the LES are not as easily accounted for. The increased sensitivity of the LES to gastrin was thought to be a significant clue to the mystery of the LES in achalasia, but the doses used in such studies have been pharmacological rather than physiological so this interesting finding is now considered insignificant in the pathophysiology of the disease.

Symptoms. Symptoms usually include significant dysphagia for liquids and solids, sometimes associated with postprandial chest pain that may mimic angina. Such pain is more common during the early phases of the disease when the pressure generated by an abnormal muscle contraction can be high. Later on, the pressures are severely dampened, and pain is unusual in contrast to the syndrome associated with SIDES, which causes significant chest pain even after years. Many authors suggest that a barium swallow and motility constitutes the mandatory investigation in patients with suspected achalasia, but I believe that the considerations presented above indicate a stronger need for endoscopy in many of these patients. Endoscopy is the only test that can discover those patients with carcinoma of the cardia mimicking achalasia.

Treatment. The treatment for achalasia is similar to that described for SIDES; pleasant surroundings, avoidance of aggravating food (often alcohol, spices, hot or cold foods), and remaining upright after meals are helpful. Although controversial, bougienage has helped some patients empty their esophagus with no need for further treatment for weeks or months. It has no permanent effect, however, and such patients will eventually require more definitive measures. These consist of pneumatic dilatation with one of the pressure-regulated bags and surgical division of esophageal musculature in the lower third (the Heller operation). The purpose of bag dilatation is to tear the musculature of the lower sphincter enabling the ineffectively contracting body of the esophagus to empty its contents unimpeded by the previously high-pressure, unyielding LES. The dilatation is achieved by one of several bags whose waist is placed with fluoroscopic guidance at the LES. Inflation pressure is limited to 300 to 500 mm Hg. The procedure nearly always causes pain and sometimes ruptures the esophagus (5 per cent). It works most of the time (80 per cent) and may be repeated once or twice. Continued failure of the method should induce consideration of surgical treatment (Bennett & Hendrix, 1970).

Heller operations for achalasia also have an 80 per cent success rate. The smooth musculature is divided from the cardia cephalad about 7 to 10 cm. In addition to the usual surgical complications associated with general anesthesia and a chest incision, the treatment can be blighted by failure to cure symptoms, severe reflux esophagitis with resultant stricture, or unrecognized, inadvertent surgical perforation of the esophagus during incision of the muscle. In spite of these ill-starred pitfalls, most patients with achalasia benefit from bag dilatation or surgical treatment, but invasive methods should be reserved for those with aspiration, weight loss, or severe symptoms warranting such imperfect "cures."

Other Considerations

One should not leave the discussion of SIDES and achalasia without recognizing that there are some patients who have features of both and some patients who have different diseases with some similar features that can cause confusion. Most motility laboratories have had referred to them patients who, upon being investigated for transport dysphagia, produce a manometric tracing with high pressure, with simultaneous waves but a normal LES, or with a high-pressure, poorly relaxing LES but normal pressure waves in the body. The treatment of these conditions is similar or identical to that of SIDES and achalasia, but physicians who are unfamiliar with them can become confused and may muddle along rendering incomplete or imprecise treatment.

Other diseases must be included when transport dysphagia is considered. Although the classic manometric abnormalities of achalasia and SIDES are not mimicked by these diseases, some features are similar. The treatment is not similar, however, so the physician should exercise precision in considering them. Patients with scleroderma (Marks, 1983) may have visceral disease, and esophageal involvement is the most common. Esophageal symptoms are present in about half the patients. Transport dysphagia may be responsible, but entrance dysphagia caused by a stricture is a possibility. The poor tone of the LES coupled with impaired acid clearance causes esophagitis in many of the patients. In fact, symptoms seem to correlate better with sphincter abnormalities than with impaired motility of the body of the esophagus (Saladin, et al., 1966).

The esophagram of the patient with scleroderma may show dilatation, impaired emptying with air fluid level, and parrot beaking at the LES. If one watches the lower esophagus, however, the reward will be opening of the LES with ultimate visual evidence that the muscle is incompetent, a finding not seen in achalasia (Fig. 1–2). Manometric data include low amplitude, simultaneous contractions in the body of the esophagus in response to swallows, and a normal or low-pressure gastroesophageal sphincter that often fails to relax during deglutition. One sees that this pattern is similar to the one observed in achalasia, particularly if the LES pressure is at the upper limit of normal in the patient with scleroderma.

Raynaud's phenomenon will nearly always be present when scleroderma involves the esophagus, a fact that led Zarafonetis (1958) to postulate a neurohumoral cause for both phenomena. The hypothesis has thus far been impossible to prove. The association between the two is clinically useful, though, and visceral scleroderma has been suspected and subsequently proved because the physician recognized the relationship and made proper investigations. All of these clinical features can be seen in lupus, dermatomyositis, and other collagen diseases, especially when Raynaud's phenomenon is present (Stevens, et al., 1964).

The importance of diagnosing this group of diseases lies in the poor response one expects from treatment. This failure is probably

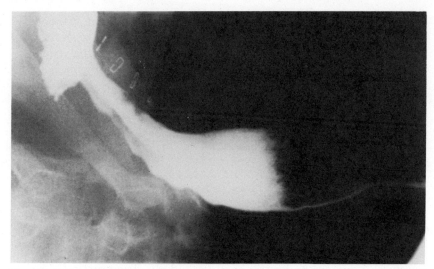

Figure 1–2. Scleroderma. In contrast to the esophagus shown in Figure 1–1, this dilated esophagus ends in an open lower esophageal sphincter whose incompetence adds to the patient's troubles. Surgical procedures to correct an accompanying hiatal hernia do not help these patients.

related to the esophagitis that so frequently complicates the primary problem. Poor acid clearance interferes with attempts at healing, and the result is a patient whose esophagus has two complicated abnormalities that cause symptoms and aggravate each other. For some time investigators also thought that adenocarcinoma was an expected complication of scleroderma, and many recommended endoscopic surveillance; but this problem, at least, has been eliminated by the studies of Segel and colleagues (1985).

The temptation to ask the surgeon to step in and slay this dragon is almost irresistible, but it must be overcome because operations are not of proven value to these patients. In fact, if the surgeon is not sophisticated and the operation includes a vagotomy, the patient may suffer the fatal complication of irreversible ileus. Even if spared this disaster, the patient may obtain no relief. The moral: if surgical treatment is being considered for one of these patients, consider all possible results carefully and share these thoughts with the patient, who is a most valuable ally in attempting to formulate the management plan.

Other diseases can cause simultaneous or low amplitude waves in the body of the esophagus in response to swallowing. One of these, originally named presbyesophagus (Khan, et al., 1977), may not exist as such. Careful evaluation (Hollis & Castell, 1974) indicates that many or most individuals whose x-rays are diagnosed as "curling" or as presbyesophagus and whose manometric studies are characterized by high-, normal-, or low-pressure simultaneous waves in response to swallowing suffer from diabetes (Stewart, et al., 1976), alcoholism, thyroid disease, esophagitis, or some other condition that could be responsible for the motility abnormality. Many such patients have no symptoms (Atkinson & Hosking, 1983), so the abnormality itself can be ignored. Instead, it serves as a guidepost that should alert the physician to consider an underlying disease (Hollis, et al., 1977).

REFLUX

Pathologic Physiology

Toothlessness and gastroesophageal reflux are common in the elderly and in newborn babies. Babies can be burped and are seldom harmed by their chalasia, but reflux may represent a real threat to the esophageal mucosa and/or lungs of the elderly. The exact relationship among hiatus hernia, esophagitis, increased intraabdominal pressure, drugs and hormones, pregnancy, adult "chalasia," sundry foods, and reflux is not fully understood. Fortunately, research continues to establish certain truths and eliminate error based upon armchair reasoning, just as Sherlock Holmes gathered the data to test the hypotheses of his brilliant but sedentary brother, Mycroft. The findings are fascinating, if sometimes confusing.

The lower esophageal sphincter is somehow a key to the reflux puzzle, but it is not the only one. The intraabdominal/intrathoracic pressure relationships are also important, and acid clearing may be the major determinant that allows or prevents mucosal damage once reflux occurs. We know for instance that normal persons, because of sphincter relaxation, experience reflux one or two times an hour (Kaye, 1977) but do not suffer from it. Patients with peptic esophagitis reflux three or four times an hour. The esophagus affected by inflammation allows more reflux and clears the acid poorly, a vicious circle (Dodds, et al., 1982). Furthermore, heartburn does not correlate quantitatively with the severity of esophagitis (Simeone, et al., 1977). In fact, stricture may occur more frequently in asymptomatic or minimally symptomatic patients.

Lower Esophageal Sphincter

Large sums of money and time have been spent in an attempt to determine the relative importance of the sphincter and the relationship of the cardia to the hiatus vis-à-vis this thorny problem of reflux. Reflux does not correlate with the pressure of the LES in an individual patient, but reflux is more common in a group of patients with low sphincter pressures than in a group with normal pressures. Barium has been observed to move from the stomach to the esophagus during various positioning maneuvers, nearly all of which are accompanied by movement of the sphincter into the thoracic cavity. The conclusion reached, particularly by surgeons, is that the presence of a hiatus hernia somehow interferes with proper operation of the LES, fostering reflux, and that such anatomical aberrations must be fixed.

Effects of Drugs on LES

Table 1–1 (Cattau & Castell, 1982) underscores the large number of substances that have an effect on the LES. The clinical importance of these is not known. Attention is drawn to the common foods that reduce the LESP and to the effect of three commonly prescribed drugs; theophylline, Valium, and verapamil. Notice the contradiction inherent in the coffee-caffeine effects. Coffee has been incriminated by many patients as a cause of heartburn. Why this is so is unclear, but the effect of coffee on the LESP seems to be related in some way to this property of causing heartburn. Those patients who suffer after the ingestion of coffee have a poor increase in LESP when compared with normals. In addition, a coffee drip causes them to report heartburn. The substance may be a primary irritant to these persons. Similar findings have been reported for orange juice even when its pH has been adjusted to neutrality (Price, et al., 1978). Notice also the effect of chocolate and a few other foods commonly incriminated by patients as the cause of their heartburn.

Other Factors

There is the additional question of the importance of acid clearance and of reduction of esophageal pH by saliva. When saliva is removed from the mouth, pH reduction is slowed, and when saliva flow is augmented by sucking on candy, alkalinization is more rapid (Helm, et al., 1984). One wonders how to use all this information.

Diagnosis

More important to the primary-care physician is the establishment of a diagnosis. Usually one has little difficulty establishing that a patient has reflux because heartburn is a well-known symptom that patients report accurately. Often enough, however, the presenting complaint is more confusing (Navab & Texter, 1985). Chest pain mimicking angina, wheezing reminiscent of asthma, cough, and dysphagia due to stricture all may have reflux as their underlying cause. Once this hurdle is overcome, the physician must still ask the right question when considering the course the investigation will take. Possible tests related to

TABLE 1–1. The Effects of Various Agents on the Lower
Esophageal Sphincter Pressure (LESP)

AGENT	EFFECT ON LESP
Hormones	
Angiotensin	+
Cholecystokinin	−
Gastric inhibitory peptide	−
Gastrin/pentagastrin	+
Glucagon	−
Motilin	+
Pancreatic polypeptide	+
Progesterone	−
Secretin	−
Substance P	+
Vasoactive intestinal polypeptide	−
Vasopressin	+
Food	
Fat	−
Chocolate	−
Ethanol	−
Peppermint	−
Neurotransmitters	
Alpha adrenergic agonist	+ or −
Anticholinergic	−
Anticholinesterase	+
Beta adrenergic agonist	−
Cholinergic agents	−
Dopamine	−
Metoclopramide	+
Miscellaneous	
Caffeine	−
Coffee	+
Demerol/morphine	−
Gastric acidification	−
Gastric alkalinization	+
Histamine	+
5-hydroxytryptamine	+
Indomethacin	+
Inflammation	−
Nitroprusside	−
Prostaglandins E, E_2, A_2, D_2	−
Prostaglandin F_{2a}	+
Protein meal	+
Theophylline	−
Valium	−
Verapamil	−

reflux include measurement of the LESP, pH testing of the lower esophagus, the acid perfusion test of Bernstein, endoscopy, x-ray examination (both routine and cine-esophagrams), radionuclide scintiscan, and acid clearing. If one wants to document the presence of reflux, a barium esophagram, scintiscan, or pH measurement of the lower esophagus when acid is present in the stomach are possible methods of examination. Barium studies are not very sensitive, but if they show reflux, one needs no further proof. The scintiscan (Fisher, et al., 1976) is sensitive and noninvasive; the pH probe is invasive but is the gold standard. Except for research problems and difficult diagnostic dilemmas, one usually skips these tests because they ordinarily do not change management.

If one must know the presence and/or extent of damage, the available tests include barium esophagram and endoscopy with biopsy (Behar & Sheahan, 1975). The latter should be performed with a suction device (Ismail-Beijr, et al., 1970), particularly when damage is not seen by gross inspection. Again, these tests are listed in increasing order of sensitivity and invasiveness.

When mechanisms are at issue, measurement of LESP and acid clearing can be useful. When the question is whether symptoms are caused by the reflux, acid perfusion tests are helpful; but because they have a subjective end-point, they are error-prone.

Although most of these tests are familiar, a brief description of the acid perfusion pH test for reflux and of scintiscan might be useful. Both acid perfusion and pH testing require the insertion of a nasogastric tube, so they are best done together. The pH probe is fixed to a tube which is used to deliver 0.1 N-HCl to the stomach for reflux testing or to the esophagus for perfusion. In the perfusion test, the acid is delivered into the lower third of the esophagus at a rate of 20 to 60 drops per minute while the patient remains sitting. If symptoms matching those being investigated appear within 20 minutes and are promptly relieved by antacid or saline flush, the test is positive. Unfortunately, the test is thought to be capable of evoking angina (Mellow, et al., 1983). After 200 ml of HCl have been placed in the stomach, the pH in the lower 5 cm of the esophagus should not drop below 5 or fall more than 2 pH units. For the scintiscan, technetium sulfur colloid is placed in the stomach. Pictures by the gamma camera show reflux much better than does a barium esophagram (Seibert, et al., 1983). Furthermore, the test can be quantitated by comparing the numbers recorded by a counter probe placed over the esophagus and then over the stomach. These tests are not needed in the usual case, but when treatment fails or clinical findings are confusing and at odds, there is security in their use.

Complications

Continuing reflux can result in stricture (Fig. 1–3), ulcer of the esophagus with or without hemorrhage, metaplasia of esophageal mucosa (Barrett's esophagus), and pulmonary disease. There is a belief

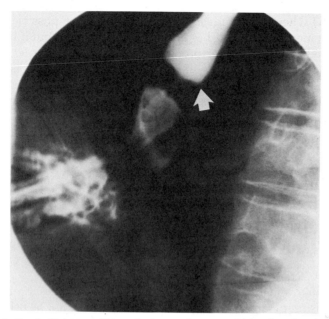

Figure 1–3. Peptic Stricture. Although the esophagus could be thought of as having a shoulder (arrow), this short concentric stricture is benign, having been caused by reflux esophagitis.

that chronic inflammation, especially when it is associated with metaplasia, increases the incidence of carcinoma (Witt, et al., 1983).

Treatment

Treatment of symptomatic reflux does not require extensive investigation in the beginning. Many patients have an episode or two of heartburn that lasts for a week or so. The symptoms are typical and the response to treatment is excellent. Most clinicians agree that these persons can be treated symptomatically and seen once or twice in follow-up to be sure that an important warning of serious underlying disease is not ignored. For those with confusing histories, poor response to treatment, or recurrent illness, a more searching evaluation should be done including one or more of the tests listed above. This is necessary to prevent or detect complications and to assure oneself and the patient that more serious diseases are absent.

Clinical Caveats

Medical management is more often successful when it includes consideration of "minor" details. Elevation of the head of the bed by means of 6-inch blocks rather than by bending the mattress helps gravity keep the gastric contents where they belong. This, along with the companion advice of eating small meals and avoiding bedtime snacks, may spell the difference between success and failure if symptoms are the end-point being considered. Weight should be normal. These maneuvers are directed toward the objective of minimizing reflux.

Attempts to increase the LESP also help stop reflux. They include avoidance of fat, e.g., chocolate, and possibly caffeine, tobacco, alcohol, anticholinergic drugs, and increased abdominal pressure. The latter relates mainly to obesity and tight clothes. Cholinergics and metoclopramide are theoretically helpful with regard to increasing LESP.

Drugs

Also considered helpful is acid reduction by means of antacids of H_2 blockers. Acid clearance is aided by Urecholine and metoclopramide. The clinical benefit of this modality is not cast in the bronze of hard proof, but the theory makes sense. Combinations of H_2 blockers and clearing agents, although logical for treatment of severe cases, are probably unwarranted (Temple, et al., 1983).

Surgical Treatment

If conservative treatment does not help, one considers surgical measures. I believe that some baseline measurement of the degree of reflux and mucosal damage is indicated before embarking on this dramatic and incondite treatment. One should be able to determine whether therapy has done any good when the bill exceeds $5,000.00. Indications for surgery include severe symptoms that respond poorly to medical therapy, bleeding, and pulmonary complications. Of these, the first is hardest to judge. Symptomatic response to a therapeutic regimen is highly subjective, another good reason for thorough evaluation of surgical candidates. Once the decision to operate is made, a dilemma remains because there are about half a dozen surgical approaches. One suspects, rightfully, that none of them is perfect or even fully acceptable. Each has its advantages, often technical, and disadvantages, often clinical.

The pre-WW II Allison repair was an attempt to re-establish normal anatomy of the diaphragmatic esophageal hiatus by suturing it to "normal" size and sewing the phrenoesophageal ligament to the diaphragm to keep the gastroesophageal junction in the abdominal cavity. The Collis modification required the additional step of anchoring the fundus of the stomach to the diaphragm. It had a radiological recurrence rate of 2.5 per cent compared with almost 50 per cent for the Allison repair. Each was blighted with a 20 per cent recurrence of symptoms.

As surgical anatomists began to understand the area better, new approaches were devised, each distinguished by a more aggressive attempt to anchor the LES below the hiatus. The Hill posterior gastropexy repairs the hiatus and anchors the lesser curve to the median arcuate ligament. Six per cent recur radiologically and 3 to 10 per cent have symptomatic failure. The Belsey Mark IV repair, a partial, anterolateral fundoplication, can be used unless the esophagus is short or strictured. It does not work if the LES slides back into the chest. Recurrence rates are 12 percent the first 3 years and 15 per cent in ten years. The Nissen fundoplication is more aggressive and effective. The wrap of the fundus is 360°, and the operation works even if the LES slides into the chest. Radiological and symptomatic recurrence rates are both 10 per cent. A simple, quick operation to combat reflux is the insertion of an Angelchik prosthesis at the lower esophagus. The device is an incomplete ring covered with Dacron so that it can be sewn into place at the cardia. It prevents reflux but tends to be rejected by the body so that about 10 per cent of them must be removed because of migration. In one series, almost 40 per cent of the patients had dysphagia postoperatively. Fortunately, the symptom was transient, and results were considered good or better in more than 90 per cent of the cases as opposed to 80 per cent in a parallel group treated by means of a Nissen fundoplication (Gear, et al., 1984). The high migration rate and its frequent requirement for removal constitute negative characteristics of this otherwise promising treatment; further evaluation is required.

There are other surgical repairs, some quite imaginative, but further discussion of such technical matters is beyond the scope of this chapter. If these operations worked well enough and were free of complications, one would be less wary of recommending them. For now, it is wise to stick to the indications mentioned above, being very careful when evaluating intractability.

INFECTIONS

Candida

Infectious diseases of the esophagus are more common than one thought in the days before fiberoptic endoscopy. One admittedly biased study from a referral center (Kodski, et al., 1976) indicated that *Candida* infection is to be found in 6 per cent of patients undergoing upper gastrointestinal endoscopy. The manifestations varied from none to overwhelming sepsis. When other gastrointestinal organs are infected by *C. albicans*, the esophagus is nearly always involved. This point is of great diagnostic importance because patients who have irritable bowel symptoms may be found to have the fungus in their stool cultures; it is a common inhabitant of the gastrointestinal tract. In the absence of esophageal invasion by the organism, one would do well to remain circumspect about a diagnosis of yeast gastroenteritis in such persons because the treatment complications could be harmful, expensive, or both. Several decades ago, clinicians thought that predisposing factors were imperative if one attempted the diagnosis of monilial esophagitis; and diabetes mellitus, cancer of the esophagus, immune disease, and indeed peptic esophagitis have been associated with it, as has the use of antibiotics. Normal persons, however, may be affected by the disease, a situation requiring the clinician to be ever alert to the possibility of this treatable condition.

Diagnosis and Differential Diagnosis

Attention is drawn to esophageal involvement in a pathological process by the complaint of dysphagia or, more characteristically, odynophagia. Since these symptoms are usually the result of organic disease, prompt investigation is required. A barium esophagram may be normal, especially if the newer techniques of double contrast and high resolution photography are not used. When the study is abnormal, the esophagram may demonstrate a shaggy esophageal wall, nodular excrescences scattered over the mucosa, one or more ulcers, filling defects caused by the luxuriant growth of the mycelium, poor emptying, or narrowing due to scar, particularly in the midesophagus where peptic stricture is less common. Sometimes the radiologist can make a fairly accurate diagnosis, but as we shall see, other diseases may mimic these findings (Eras, et al., 1972). Therefore, an endoscopy will be requested in most cases. The endoscopist will see erythema with a grey membrane distributed in a patchy arrangement that may spare the lower few centimeters of the esophagus. If the membrane is wiped, the undersurface is friable and bleeds easily. Sometimes the distribution is more universal causing even more difficulty in differentiating it from peptic esophagitis. Endoscopists do not culture the lesion because C. albicans can be found in the esophagus normally. Biopsy is useful to exclude other lesions such as herpes, but the best procedure is brushing and preparation of a slide so that yeast forms can be sought under the microscope. These tests may be negative in the presence of disease. This is unfortunate because some of the infections described below can imitate candidiasis, and one dislikes empirical treatment under these circumstances. Serological tests will not help because they may be positive in the absence of disease and negative in its presence. The differential diagnosis lies mainly between candidiasis and one of the following: severe reflux, herpes esophagitis, lactobacillus invasion, or infection with *Torulopsis glabrata*. Severe reflux esophagitis usually does not have the tenaciously adherent exudate with bleeding undersurface seen in *Candida* infection. Unfortunately, *C. albicans* may superinfect an esophagus injured by acid or bile reflux, a source of confusion in the diagnosis. Herpes and *Candida* infections may be differentiated by examining the material in the border of the lesions for the cellular inclusions and multinucleated giant cells so characteristic of herpes infection.

Treatment

Treatment with a viscous suspension of nystatin (Kantrowitz, 1969) has been effective if cumbersome. Systemic use of amphotericin B has been useful in stubborn cases, particularly those associated with mucocutaneous candidiasis. A convenient and apparently safe treatment is with ketoconazole in a dosage of 200 mg daily for 8 days. The tablets are easy to take, and the drug's effectiveness is perfectly acceptable when compared with other treatments (Fazio, et al., 1983). Because ketoconazole is chemically similar to metronidazole, the two share metronidazole's Antabuse-like reaction to alcohol ingestion.

Herpetic Esophagitis

Frequently missed because it causes few symptoms, herpetic esophagitis (Fishbein, et al., 1979) is not as rare in adults as clinicians believe. An autopsy review at the Bowman Gray School of Medicine (Buss & Scharyj, 1979) established the presence of herpes infection of the esophagus in 50 of 56 cases manifesting visceral infection. In 41 cases, the esophagus was the only organ involved. Most of these patients had no esophageal symptoms during their lifetimes. Malignant neoplasms were present in 34 patients; of these 14 were carcinomas, the rest were leukemia, lymphoma, or multiple myeloma. Serious, nonmalignant disease or trauma was associated with 19 others. About 60 per cent were men averaging 57 years of age, the usual age and sex mix for autopsies at Bowman Gray.

Because specific treatment for such cases has been limited, clinicians have concentrated their diagnostic thinking on other diseases, especially candidiasis, with which herpes can be confused. Examination of biopsies of the margins of the discrete ulcers found in the esophageal mucosa shows inclusions in the epithelial cells and the presence of multinucleated giant cells. The ulcers, particularly when they are large, are easily infected by secondary invaders including bacteria and fungus. If the fungus is *C. albicans*, more diagnostic confusion is certain. Fortunately, these patients do not die of the disease. One suspects, however, that some may die because of it. Investigators have postulated that the ulcers may serve as portals of entry for the bacteria and fungi that grow in them. The results of dissemination, especially in the usual immunocompromised host harboring the herpetic infection, are disastrous. The onus of diagnosis clearly falls on the gastroenterologist since the esophagus is involved in almost 90 per cent of cases (Matsumoto & Sumiyoshi, 1985).

Other Infections

Lactobacillus acidophilus

Not uncommonly, one is confronted by cases of "monilial esophagitis" whose esophageal samples fail to yield microscopic or culture evidence of the presence of C. albicans. Surely some of these cases represent another disease, and a report from Edinburgh (McManus & Webb, 1975) suggests Lactobacillus acidophilus as one candidate. An esophageal lesion that was thought to be caused by monilia manifested no mycelia or yeast forms. Instead, there flourished a mass of gram-positive rods and leukocytes that when cultured yielded L. acidophilus. Although the organism was by in vitro tests sensitive to tetracycline, the patient did not respond symptomatically or endoscopically and ultimately died of her valvular heart disease. Postmortem examination confirmed the previous endoscopic and biopsy findings. Even though the example illustrated by this case does not fulfill Koch's postulates, one would do well to keep it in mind when presented with monilial esophagitis that does not yield C. albicans on microscopic examination.

Torulopsis glabrata

Also thought originally to be a commensal organism, Torulopsis glabrata has been implicated in esophageal infections. The fungus closely resembles C. albicans, and the authors (Bentlif & Wiedermann, 1979) of the case report, which suggested it as a cause of esophagitis, believed that their patients may have had a predisposing factor as is often the case in moniliasis. The esophagoscopic findings were similar to those of moniliasis. Treatment with Mycostatin is probably effective, so confusion with candidiasis does not cause serious consequences.

NEOPLASMS

When dealing with patients in the older age group, the physician is always sensitive to the specter of neoplasm as a cause of symptoms. Esophageal symptoms are no exception. Furthermore, benign neoplasm of the esophagus is rare compared with the rather high incidence of carcinoma of the organ.

Benign Growths

Leiomyoma

Leiomyoma is probably the most familiar benign tumor of the esophagus. It is less rare than some others described below, but because it frequently causes no symptoms, it may be found by accident or at postmortem examination. Symptomatic or not, when a mass is found in a patient, one is faced with decisions. Should there be further investigation? Is surgical removal indicated? What follow-up is required? Sometimes, these simple questions require difficult answers.

Treatment

If symptoms are annoying, the patient will solve the problem by demanding relief. When they are absent, anxiety of the patient or the doctor may be the overriding indication for removal. The tumor appears by roentgen examination to be an intramural, extramucosal lesion; this can be confirmed by endoscopy, but one often wonders about sarcomatous degeneration, and biopsies are not helpful because they do not sample the tumor adequately. The confident and intrepid patient and physician will watch the lesion by means of serial esophagrams. If it enlarges, removal is recommended. The operation is relatively simple because esophagectomy will seldom be required; the tumor shells out easily most of the time.

Lipoma

Occurring with increasing frequency as the gastrointestinal tract proceeds aborally, lipomas of the gut usually arise from the submucosa. These rare tumors grow to a large size before they produce symptoms. Esophageal lipomas usually have a narrow stalk that originates at the pharyngoesophageal junction. This anatomical feature is responsible for the principal danger of this easily removable tumor—death by aspiration (Allen & Talbot, 1967). Unfortunately, such an incident may be the initial manifestation of an esophageal lipoma, but occasionally a patient will have regurgitated the fleshy mass into the mouth and swallowed it without consulting a physician. Because this is such a rare event, it may be misinterpreted even if the physician learns of it. Such errors are unfortunate since the tumor can be removed by endoscopic means.

Squamous Papillomas

Squamous papillomas of the esophagus are rare too. Because of this, management is unclear. Less than 20 have been reported, most in men, about half of whom have complained of dysphagia. The tumors usually have been treated by endoscopic removal. Since the relationship of these benign tumors to future malignancy is unknown, there is uncertainty about whether or not to remove asymptomatic ones. Squamous papillomas originating elsewhere have been considered premalignant, however, so removal when feasible is currently recommended (Zeabart, 1979).

Lymphangiomas

Although lymphangiomas of the esophagus may mimic leiomyomas because they appear to be intramural and extramucosal when seen on an esophagram, their esophagoscopic appearance will differ. The tumor is compressible and translucent. Biopsy removed by means of the forceps used with fiberoptic esophagoscopes may be inadequate for diagnosis, but a large specimen obtained through a rigid esophagoscope made the diagnosis in a case reported by Brady and Milligan (1973)—the luck of the Irish? The disease is so rare that one will be lucky to suspect it.

Others

Epithelial cysts and *fibrovascular polyps* likewise are rare, as are *inflammatory pseudotumors* (LiVolsi & Perzin, 1975). The latter also mimic leiomyomas, but they are sometimes pedunculated. They are located at or near the Z line where they can also be confused with carcinoma. Biopsy is indicated; it will usually solve the problem (Styles, et al., 1985).

Malignancies

Squamous Cell Carcinoma

Much more common and lethal is carcinoma of the esophagus, which is the sixth most common gastrointestinal malignancy in the United States (Silverberg & Lubera, 1986). It is even more common in China and in Russia where the incidence is 130 and 51/100,000 population, respectively, compared with 4/100,000 in the United States and Great Britain (Swarbrick, 1985). One should be more alert to its presence in patients who smoke and drink excessively or who have had head and neck cancer. Of less importance but noteworthy are a history of lye stricture, a history of radiation treatment involving the esophagus, achalasia, and reflux especially when accompanied by Barrett's epithelium.

Symptoms

Dysphagia is a symptom that is usually associated with organic disease. It should be investigated promptly particularly when the epidemiological features described above are present. In the elderly, carcinoma will often be found during such investigations, which should include endoscopy when any doubt arises. One of the major problems associated with esophageal carcinoma is the advanced stage of disease at the time of diagnosis. Poor prognosis can be expected under these circumstances. By the time pain is an important complaint, the outlook is dim indeed because the symptom indicates local extension. The absence of a serosal layer around the esophagus may be the principal reason for early spread of cancer of the organ. In addition, dysphagia requires a major obstruction of the lumen since the esophagus is a distensible organ; even experienced gastroenterologists are amazed at the collection of items that have been swallowed by the insane. At least dysphagia will alert the physician to think of the esophagus. Chest pain may be more confusing early in its course. Anorexia and weight loss are even less specific but no less important. Gastrointestinal hemorrhage is brisk less than 5 per cent of the time, but slow bleeding resulting in anemia is common. Because the recurrent laryngeal nerve approximates the esophagus for some of its course, hoarseness can be the presenting symptom of these patients. A similar anatomical fact—apposition of the esophagus, trachea, and aorta—accounts for occasional tracheoesophageal fistulae or erosion of the tumor into the aorta with a rapid, dramatic death.

An occasional patient will manifest the nephrotic syndrome caused by membranous glomerulonephritis (Heckerling, 1985) or will exhibit some other paraneoplastic syndrome.

Metastases

Carcinoma of the esophagus spreads locally to surrounding mediastinal structures, lymph nodes, lung, and pericardium. Distant visceral involvement is most common in liver and lung, but other viscera can be attacked. Aspiration pneumonitis caused by tracheoesophageal fistula or obstruction is found in about half the cases examined by autopsy.

Diagnosis and Staging

Ordinarily, the diagnosis is easy—too easy—but it can be illusive indeed (Walfish, et al., 1985). The radiologist who is informed of the clinician's suspicions will make special efforts to turn the patient into various positions in an attempt to demonstrate lesions of the anterior or posterior esophageal walls that could be obscured by the barium column in an anteroposterior projection. Endoscopy with biopsy, cytology, or both is required for a tissue diagnosis. If the lesion is located near the cricopharyngeus or at the cardia, one may have more difficulty demonstrating it.

In an attempt to avoid a major thoracic operation for an incurable patient, one should stage those patients who are being considered for surgical treatment. Bronchoscopy and mediastinoscopy have been considered important in this regard, but the introduction of CT scanning may also have made an important contribution for this purpose (Schneekloth, et al., 1983). The noninvasive CT scan of the chest and upper abdomen can demonstrate local (Fig. 1–4) or widespread metastases in the chest or liver and can eliminate the need for further investigation or for consideration of surgical treatment (Fig. 1–5). Since most of these patients smoke, they are frequently bad surgical risks because of accompanying lung disease. Detractors of CT staging have made their appearance (Lea, et al., 1984), so one would do well to follow the literature about this staging method.

Treatment

General Considerations
After all these factors have been considered, one is faced with controversy about the value of various forms of therapy in the different thirds of the esophagus. Standard wisdom dictates surgical treatment

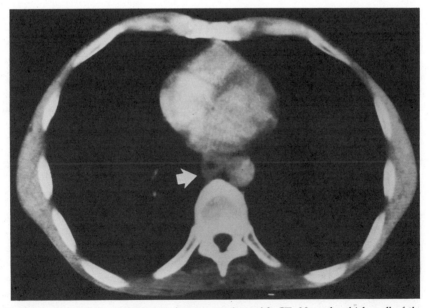

Figure 1–4. Carcinoma of the esophagus—staging with CT. Note the thick wall of the esophagus as it lies in close apposition to the aorta. It takes little imagination to conjure up an image of this tumor eroding through the aortic wall with dramatic, disastrous results.

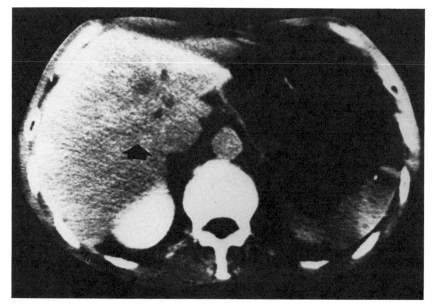

Figure 1–5. Staging esophageal cancer. The liver of the same patient shown in Figure 1–4 exhibits metastases (arrow) later proved by aspiration. A major operation may be avoided by proper application of this noninvasive test.

for lesions of the lower third and irradiation for those of the upper third. Carcinoma of the middle third is thrown to the wolves, presumably being treated by the physician or surgeon with the greatest panache. Launois, et al., (1983) were able to resect 70 per cent of the esophageal carcinomas in a series of 360 patients. Half of the 34 upper third lesions fell prey to the knife. The 5-year survival rate of the whole cadre was only 5 per cent. One wonders whether the price—18 per cent mortality and 12 per cent anastomotic leak—is too high especially if irradiation treatment is comparable in terms of discomfort and cost as well as results.

Surgical

The Chinese (Xu, et al., 1983), who see more cancer of the esophagus, report higher resectability rates and lower surgical mortality (10 per cent) and complication rates in all three sections of esophagus— a different disease there? The 5-year survival rate of 22 per cent is more promising. In 1984, my own hospital's tumor registry reported 17 cases of esophageal carcinoma; 16 were treated surgically for cure, but at the operating table, 5 had local and 9 had regional metastases. One was a carcinoma in situ. This common experience underscores the usual resistant problem faced by patients and their physicians in the United States.

Radiotherapy

Radiotherapy for cure (Pearson, 1977) results in a 3 to 10 per cent 5-year survival rate, but a series of 99 treated in Edinburgh (Pearson, 1974) resulted in 20 5-year survivors. Palliative irradiation is employed more commonly and with some benefit. Symptoms are frequently relieved for months or even a year or two. Whether the addition or substitution of chemotherapy is useful is not known. Those engaged in it should have wide experience so that they can interpret the results.

Palliation

The matter of palliation is of great importance because cure is so unlikely. The physician's first duty is to relieve suffering. Because dysphagia is the most common symptom of recurrent or untreated but incurable cancer of the esophagus, dilatation of the narrowed lumen is a frequent palliative procedure. Bougienage is often used because it is effective and easy to do. If the stricture is very tight or the lumen is eccentric, the danger is greater. The cautious physician will then use a guide wire to ensure that the dilating instrument follows the correct path through the tumor. Whether a metal olive, balloon, or tapered device is used is a technical matter to be left to the operator; a tapered device (Dumon, et al., 1985) or balloon would seem safer.

Celestin Tube. Unfortunately, strictures tend to recur, and a gastrostomy, which is good for nutrition, will not take care of oral secretions. A Celestin tube (Carter & Hinshaw, 1963) is a prosthesis that can be inserted across the length of the tumor to combat this problem. Seated permanently, it allows the remaining weeks or months to be free of the misery of spitting oral secretions and can also be used to seal a tracheoesophageal fistula. Originally, the devices were placed surgically. Later, they were seated using a bougie and pusher tube. Now more elaborate kits are available, but they still use the principles so well described by Peura and colleagues (1978). The funnel-shaped device is seated with its flange above the carcinoma and its stem across the narrowed area. If the tumor is high in the esophagus, the flange may seat near the cricopharyngeus causing gagging or aspiration. Such a tumor location is, therefore, a contraindication to the use of the Celestin tube or other such devices.

Laser. More recently, endoscopists with laser experience have used neodymium:yttrium-aluminum-garnet (Nd:YAG) laser to carve out the lumen through the tumor (Mellow & Pinkas, 1985). The procedure is easy and safe in experienced hands but does not always result in relief of symptoms. However, for the 70 per cent of cases in whom it works, it is useful; and I have been personally pleased the few times I have referred patients to the "laser doctor" for help with this problem.

Adenocarcinoma

Adenocarcinoma can arise from the esophagus because of its mucous glands, but it accounts for less than 1 per cent of esophageal cancer. If Barrett's esophagus is included, the figure may reach 3 per cent. Controversy continues about whether or not these lesions actually arise from the cardia of the stomach, but the argument makes little difference clinically. The lesions are suspected and diagnosed using the same principles described for squamous cell carcinoma, and the prognosis is just as miserable. It has been widely believed that such histological types of carcinoma do not respond to irradiation, although a study from Copenhagan (Cederqvist, et al., 1980) refutes that notion.

Barrett's Esophagus

Barrett's esophagus is worth considering separately because esophagologists are beginning to solidify an opinion that it is a surgical disease. This opinion is based upon follow-up of a limited number of patients with columnar metaplasia of the esophageal mucosa (Spechler, et al., 1984). For example, Starnes and colleagues (1984) culled from 439 patients with esophagitis, 40 with Barrett's epithelial change. Almost 40 per cent of these had adenocarcinoma. Of the 25 patients with no malignancy, 20 were considered to have had adequate medical treatment, yet 80 per cent of these developed a stricture or ulcer of the esophagus. The recommendation that resulted from their experience was to perform a Nissen fundoplication on patients with Barrett's esophagus and to examine them endoscopically every 6 months, checking the mucosa for dysplasia, which, if found, would constitute an indication for resection of the diseased part of the esophagus.

Witt and colleagues (1983) looked at the problem from the other perspective. They examined the material from 594 patients with esophageal carcinoma and found 19 who had Barrett's esophagus. Although 15 were resected for cure, the median survival was only a year.

Skinner (1983) has looked at these data and 43 of his own cases of Barrett's esophagus. Finding 20 malignancies in the group, he too recommended that all such persons be offered surgical treatment with endoscopic biopsy follow-up every 6 months. Such aggressive advice will be met with awe or perhaps even disbelief in some quarters, but the high incidence of fatal cancers in these patients challenges disbelievers to construct a better plan. Perhaps a study of simple lavage and cytology of a group with Barrett's esophagus would offer a less expensive, equally effective solution. Metaplasia should be suspected when the endoscopist sees a velvet-like mucosa with a red hue different from the normal pink esophageal mucosa. Biopsy will confirm the presence of metaplasia. The use of double contrast radiography may make screening for Barrett's esophagus easier and may result in earlier case finding (Levine, et al., 1983). This group recognized an unusual reticular pattern when examining the esophagus by the double contrast technique; the pattern appeared to be specific for Barrett's esophagus.

Other Malignancies

Carcinosarcoma is worth knowing about. It is polypoid so it can be confused with fibrovascular polyps and other benign lesions. It is less aggressive than squamous carcinoma or adenocarcinoma and should be treated surgically. Verrucous squamous cell carcinomas are also more indolent than the usual varieties.

Malignant melanomas are usually polypoid too. Pedunculated, these primary melanomas differ grossly from the umbilicated nodules characteristic of melanomas metastatic to the gastrointestinal tract, but they rarely arise in the esophagus.

Occasionally, a patient with adrenocorticotropic hormone (ACTH) excess, hypercalcemia, or some other endocrine abnormality, will have an *argyrophil cell carcinoma* of the esophagus. Similar histologically to an oat cell carcinoma of the lungs, these tumors also cause early death.

Metastatic cancer may also deposit and grow in the esophagus. Most frequently, this is due to invasion by a contiguous tumor of the lung or thyroid, but lymphoma and other malignancies may be responsible. Rarely, lymphoma can also arise in the esophagus.

CONCLUSION

Esophageal disease in the geriatric age group is similar to that in the younger patient; the treatment emphasis is different. Motility disorders are more likely to be related to degenerative diseases than to achalasia or SIDES, and transfer dysphagia is more common in the elderly because of this. Fungal infections are also more common in the elderly than in the young. Cancer is a prime cause of esophageal symptoms and dominates differential diagnoses in this group.

Because of these considerations, delays for therapeutic trials should be short and follow-up more careful. The endoscope must be used earlier and more often. Treatment considerations must include more thought about drug interactions and the ability of the patient to withstand surgical therapy.

Congenital diseases are infrequent; however, rings and webs must be included in diagnostic deliberations. This chapter did not mention some of these abnormalities. Schatzki rings, for example, were not described even though they occur in older people. They cause a characteristic syndrome of entrance dysphagia that is intermittent and often specific for foods such as roast beef or steak. Therefore, the appellation "steakhouse syndrome" has been applied to it.

In considering all of the things described in the chapter, I am struck with the ability to master the management of transfer dysphagia as the hallmark of a geriatric esophagologist. Caused so often by degenerative disease of the nervous system, transfer abnormalities present a challenge that is difficult to meet. Research in the care and rehabilitation of patients with central nervous system diseases must continue to address this problem because the present solutions are incomplete. Nutrition can be maintained, but the difficulties with handling secretions have not been solved. Aspiration continues to cause hospitalization and long stays for older patients, resulting in an unacceptable amount of suffering and high costs for the care of these patients.

REFERENCES

Allen, M.S., Jr., and Talbot, W.H.: Sudden death due to regurgitation of a pedunculated esophageal lipoma. J Thorac Cardiovasc Surg 54:756–758, 1967.

Arndorfer, R.C., et al: Improved infusion system for intraluminal esophageal manometry. Gastroenterology 73:23, 1977.

Atkinson, M., and Hosking, D.J.: Gastrointestinal complications of diabetes mellitus. Clin Gastroenterol 12:636, 1983.

Behar, J., and Sheahan, D.C.: Histologic abnormalities in reflux esophagitis. Arch Pathol 99:387, 1975.

Benjamin, S.B., et al.: Prospective manometric evaluation with pharmacologic provocation of patients with suspected esophageal motility dysfunction. Gastroenterology 84:893–901, 1983.

Bennett, J.R., and Hendrix, T.R.: Treatment of achalasia with pneumatic dilatation. Mod Treatment 7:1217–1228, 1970.

Bentlif, P.S., and Wiedermann, B.: Esophagitis caused by Torulopsis glabrata. Am J Gastroenterol 71:395–397, 1979.

Brady, P.G., and Milligan, F.D.: Lymphangioma of the esophagus—diagnosis by endoscopic biopsy. Dig Dis 18:423–425, 1973.

Buss, D.H., and Scharyj, M.: Herpesvirus infection of the esophagus and other visceral organs in adults. Am J Med 66:457–462, 1979.

Carter, R., and Hinshaw, D.B.: Use of the Celestin indwelling plastic tube for inoperable carcinoma of the esophagus and cardia. Surg Gynecol Obstet 117:641–644, 1963.

Cattau, E.L., and Castell, D.O.: Symptoms of esophageal dysfunction. Adv Intern Med 27:151, 1982.

Cederqvist, C., et al.: Adenocarcinoma of the esophagus. Acta Chir Scand 146:411–415, 1980.

Clause, R.E., and Lustman, P.J.: Psychiatric illness and contraction abnormalities of the esophagus. N Engl J Med 309:1337–1342, 1983.

Clause, R.E., et al.: Manometric findings during spontaneous chest pain in patients with presumed esophageal "spasm." Gastroenterology 85:395–402, 1983.

Code, C.F., et al.: An Atlas of Esophageal Motility in Health and Disease. Springfield, IL., Charles C. Thomas, 1958.

Cotzias, G.C., et al.: Modification of parkinsonism—chronic treatment with L-dopa. N Engl J Med 280:337–345, 1969.

Dodds, W.J., et al.: Mechanisms of gastroesophageal reflux in patients with reflux esophagitis. N Engl J Med 307:1547–1552, 1982.

Dumon, J., et al.: A new method of esophageal dilation using Savary-Gilliard bougies. Gastrointest Endosc 31:379–382, 1985.

Eras, P., et al.: *Candida* infection of the gastrointestinal tract. Medicine 51:367–379, 1972.

Fazio, R., et al.: Ketoconazole treatment of *Candida* esophagitis—A prospective study of 12 cases. Am J Gastroenterol 78:261–264, 1983.

Fischer, R.A., et al.: Esophageal motility in neuromuscular disorders. Ann Intern Med 63:229–248, 1965.

Fishbein, P., et al.: Herpes simplex esophagitis. Dig Dis Sci 24:540, 1979.

Fisher, R.S., et al.: Gastroesophageal (GE) scintiscanning to detect and quantitate GE reflux. Gastroenterology 70:301–313, 1976.

Gear, M.W.L., et al.: Randomized prospective trial of the Angelchik antireflux prosthesis. Br J Surg 71:681–683, 1984.

Heckerling, P.S.: Esophageal carcinoma with membranous nephropathy. Ann Intern Med 103:474, 1985.

Helm, J.F., et al.: Effect of esophageal emptying and saliva on clearance of acid from the esophagus. N Engl J Med 310:284–288, 1984.

Hollis, J.B., and Castell, D.O.: Esophageal function in elderly men. A new look at "presbyesophagus." Ann Intern Med 80:371–374, 1974.

Hollis, J.B., et al.: Esophageal function in diabetes mellitus and its relation to peripheral neuropathy. Gastroenterology 73:1098–1102, 1977.

Ismail-Beijr, F., et al.: Histological consequences of gastroesophageal reflux in man. Gastroenterology 58:163, 1970.

Kantrowitz, P., et al.: Successful treatment of chronic esophageal moniliasis with a viscous suspension of nystatin. Gastroenterology 57:424–429, 1969.

Kaye, M.D.: Post-prandial gastroesophageal reflux in healthy people. Gut 18:709, 1977.

Khan, T.A., et al.: Esophageal motility in the elderly. J Dig Dis 22:1049–1054, 1977.

Kodski, B.E., et al.: *Candida* esophagitis. Gastroenterology 71:715, 1976.

Kraft, A.R., et al.: Achalasia of the esophagus complicated by varices and massive hemorrhage. N Engl J Med 288:405–406, 1973.

Kramer, P., and Ingelfinger, F.J.: Motility of the human esophagus in control subjects and in patients with esophageal disorders. Am J Med 7:168, 1949.

Launois, B., et al.: Results of surgical treatment of carcinoma of the esophagus. Surg Gynecol Obstet 156:753, 1983.

Lea, J.W., IV, et al.: The questionable role of computed tomography in preoperative staging of esophageal cancer. Ann Thorac Surg 38:479–481, 1984.

Levine, M.S., et al.: Barrett's esophagus: Reticular pattern of the mucosa. Radiology 147:663–667, 1983.

LiVolsi, V.A., and Perzin, K.H.: Inflammatory pseudotumors (inflammatory fibrous polyps) of the esophagus. Dig Dis 20:475–481, 1975.

Mandelstane, P., and Lieber, A.: Esophageal dysfunction in diabetic neuropathy-gastropathy. JAMA 201:88–92, 1967.

Marks, J.: The relationship of gastrointestinal disease and the skin. Clin Gastroenterol 12:693, 1983.

Matsumoto, J., and Sumiyoshi, A.: Herpes simplex esophagitis—A study in autopsy series. Am J Clin Pathol 84:96–99, 1985.

McManus, J.P.A., and Webb, J.N.: A yeast-like infection of the esophagus caused by *Lactobacillus acidophilus*. Gastroenterology 68:583–586, 1975.

Mellow, M.H., and Pinkas, H.: Endoscopic laser therapy for malignancies affecting the esophagus and gastroesophageal junction. Arch Intern Med 145:1443–1446, 1985.

Mellow, M.H., et al.: Esophageal acid perfusion in coronary artery disease: Indication of myocardial ischemia. Gastroenterology 85:306–312, 1983.

Navab, F., and Texter, E.C., Jr.: Gastroesophageal reflux. Arch Intern Med 145:329–333, 1985.

Pearson, J.G.: The present status and future potential of radiotherapy in the management of esophageal cancer. Cancer 39:882, 1977.

Pearson, J.G.: Value of radiation therapy in cancer of the esophagus. JAMA 227:181, 1974.

Pelemans, W., and Vantrappen, G.: Esophageal disease in the elderly. Clin Gastroenterol 14:635–656, 1985.

Peura, D.A., et al.: Esophageal prosthesis in cancer. Dig Dis 23:796–800, 1978.

Price, C.F., et al.: Food sensitivity in reflux esophagitis. Gastroenterology 75:240, 1978.

Richter, J.E., et al.: Edrophonium: A useful provocative test for esophageal chest pain. Ann Intern Med 103:14–20, 1985.

Richter, J.E., et al.: Effects of oral calcium blocker, diltiazem on esophageal contractions: Studies in volunteers and patients with nutcracker esophagus. Dig Dis Sci 29:649–656, 1984.

Saladin, T.A., et al.: Esophageal motor abnormalities in scleroderma and related diseases. Am J Dig Dis 11:522–535, 1966.

Schneekloth, G., et al.: Computed tomography in carcinoma of esophagus and cardia. Gastrointest Radiol 8:193–206, 1983.

Segel, M. C., et al.: Systemic sclerosis (scleroderma) and esophageal adenocarcinoma: Is increased patient screening necessary? Gastroenterology 89:485–488, 1985.

Seibert, J.J., et al.: Gastroesophageal reflux—the acid test: Scintography or pH probe. Am J Roentgenol 140:1087–1090, 1983.

Silverberg, E., and Lubera, J.: Cancer statistics. CA 36:9, 1986.

Simeone, J.F., et al.: Aperistalsis and esophagitis. Radiology 123:9–14, 1977.

Skinner, D.B., et al.: Barrett's esophagus: Comparison of benign and malignant cases. Ann Surg 198:554–566, 1983.

Sleisenger, M.H., and Fordtran, J.S.: Gastrointestinal Disease: Pathophysiology Diagnosis Management. 3rd Ed, Vol 1. Philadelphia, W.B. Saunders Company, 1983, p. 439.

Spechler, S.J., et al.: Adenocarcinoma and Barrett's esophagus. An overrated risk? Gastroenterology 87:927–933, 1984.

Starnes, V.A., et al.: Barrett's esophagus: Surgical entity. Arch Surg 119:563, 1984.

Stevens, M.B., et al.: Aperistalsis of the esophagus in patients with connective tissue disorders and Raynaud's phenomenon. N Engl J Med 270:1218–1222, 1964.

Stewart, I.M., et al.: Esophageal motor changes in diabetes mellitus. Thorax 31:278–283, 1976.

Styles, R.A., et al.: Esophagogastric polyps: Radiographic and endoscopic findings. Radiology 154:307–311, 1985.

Swarbrick, E.T.: Comment, Endoscopic surveillance in *Current Medical Literature*. Gastroenterology 4:109–113, 1985.

Temple, J.G., et al.: Cimetidine and metoclopramide in esophageal reflux disease. Br Med J 1:1863–1864, 1983.

Traube, M., et al.: Effects of nifedipine in achalasia and in patients with high-amplitude peristaltic esophageal contractions. JAMA 252:1733–1736, 1984.

van Overbeck, J.J.M.: The Hypopharyngeal Diverticulum. Amsterdam, Van Goruum Assen, 1977, p. 92.

Walfish, P., et al.: Esophageal carcinoma masquerading as recurrent acute suppurative thyroiditis. Arch Intern Med 145:346–347, 1985.

Witt, T.R., et al.: Adenocarcinoma in Barrett's esophagus. J Thorac Cardiovasc Surg 85:337, 1983.

Xu, L., et al.: Surgical treatment of carcinoma of the esophagus and cardiac portion of the stomach in 850 patients. Ann Thorac Surg 35:542, 1983.

Zarafonetis, C.J.D., et al.: Association of functioning carcinoid syndrome and scleroderma. 1 case report. Am J Med Sci 236:1, 1958.

Zeabart, L., et al.: Squamous papilloma of the esophagus. Gastrointest Endosc 25:18–20, 1979.

REFERENCES FOR FURTHER READING

Berk, J.E., et al. (eds.): Bockus Gastroenterology. 4th Ed. Vol 2. Philadelphia, W.B. Saunders Company, 1985.

Connell, A.M. (ed.): Motility and its disturbances. Clin Gastroenterol 11:437–686, 1982.

Demling, L., et al.: Endoscopy and Biopsy of the Esophagus and Stomach. Philadelphia, W.B. Saunders Company, 1972, p. 12.

Horwitz, A.L., et al.: Disorders of Esophageal Motility. *In* Smith L.H., Jr. (ed.): Major Problems in Internal Medicine. Vol XVI. Philadelphia, W.B. Saunders Company, 1979.

Sleisenger, M.H., and Fordtran, J.S.: Gastrointestinal Disease: Pathophysiology, Diagnosis, Management. 3rd Ed. Philadelphia, W.B. Saunders Company, 1983.

Spiro, H.: Clinical Gastroenterology. 3rd Ed. New York, Macmillan Publishing Co., Inc., 1983.

Chapter 2
THE STOMACH

Thomas A. Saladin

Old stomachs should evoke respect from physicians; these organs must have served their owners well or neither would be old. Simply being around for a long time, however, exposes a stomach to the risk of developing degenerative diseases and malfunction, particularly when maintenance has been neglected.

A brief reminder of some anatomical and physiological principles will help increase understanding of the diseases to be described. The stomach begins at the "Z" line, located at the end of the esophagus. The 2 cm collar of mucosa just beyond the Z line is the cardia of the stomach. The glands of this area—the cardiac glands—contain cells similar to the mucous neck cells and the epithelial cells of the pylorus. The body of the stomach continues from the distal margin of the cardia to the pylorus, marked proximally by the incisura, a fairly constant fold on the lesser curvature about midway between the esophagus and the duodenum. The conical pouch where the stomach extends cephalad between the cardia and the greater curvature is called the fundus. Gastric glands in the body and fundus are composed of chief (zymogen) cells that secrete pepsinogen I and II, oxyntic (parietal) cells that secrete hydrochloric acid and intrinsic factor, mucous neck cells (few in number), and endocrine cells. Pyloric glands are made up of gastrin-secreting cells (G cells), enterochromoffin cells, and argentaffin cells. No acid is secreted by the pyloric mucosa.

Acid is secreted in response to a variety of complex, interrelated, hormonal and nervous stimuli; paracrine activity may also be involved. Protection against damage by the acid is afforded by mucus and by cellular activities whose mechanisms of action are just being explored.

The net result is a storage organ of variable capacity where digestion is begun and where entry into the rest of the intestinal milieu is modulated by complex and incompletely understood mixing and emptying activities. For example, liquids are emptied faster than solids, protein and carbohydrates faster than fats, and isosmotic material faster than hyperosmotic.

For nearly every anatomical and physiological fact, there seems to be a disease, but most are not common and few are peculiar to old age per se. Age sometimes affects the way the patient comes to the attention of the physician, however, and that is one reason for this and its fellow chapters.

CONGENITAL ANOMALIES

Given to early detection because of a predilection to announce their presence by early and attention-getting symptoms, congenital abnormalities are seldom hidden until old age. When this does happen, they may be found by accident during investigation of an unrelated symptom or at autopsy.

INFLAMMATION

Gastritis is common, if not well understood. It may be classified as erosive, nonerosive (including atrophic gastritis), hyperplastic (Ménétrier's disease), eosinophilic, or infectious. Superficial gastritis of the antrum and fundus is said to occur in 50 per cent of stomachs after the fourth decade. The significance of this finding is unknown in spite of many investigations during decades of research.

Erosive gastritis may announce its presence by a major gastrointestinal hemorrhage during the course of some other disease or may be found during a gastroscopic examination indicated for other reasons. When the condition causes hemorrhage, actions to be taken are acceptably clear and risk factors may be obvious, even if pathophysiology and pathogenesis are not. The risk factors include sepsis, renal failure, jaundice, old age, shock, and central nervous system catastrophies (Sleisenger & Fordtran, 1983). All of these conditions are serious; how they cause erosive gastritis is only partially understood. Acid must be involved in some of these risk factors because maintaining the gastric pH above 5.5 reduces by 50 per cent the incidence of bleeding from erosive gastritis. Given the fact that gastric acid secretion decreases with age, one wonders about the importance of other, particularly cellular, factors in this disease. Proof is hard to get.

Questions have been raised about the reversibility of gastritis; the possibility is suggested by studies of biopsies taken serially from dozens of patients. Some of these studies indicated return to normal in at least a few of the cases of nonspecific, nonerosive gastritis. Sampling bias could have accounted for such findings, but actual regression of disease is just as reasonable (Sleisenger & Fordtran, 1983).

Although not specifically and directly related to age, *Campylobacter pylori* is now a putative cause of type B gastritis, the kind that is seen most often in the antrum of the stomach. The story of the development of scientific thinking about the connection of this organism with pathologic change in the gastric mucosa spans 100 years (Hazell & Graham, 1988). During the past decade or two, however, researchers (Warren & Marshall, 1983) have identified, cultured, and linked *C. pylori* with several diseases of the stomach and duodenum including ulcer and gastritis. Experts have disagreed about whether *C. pylori* is *the* cause of gastritis, *a* cause of gastritis, or a secondary invader of the mucosa afflicted with gastritis, but it is now considered the principal cause of antral gastritis. The gastritis evolves from an acute inflammatory process to a chronic one, followed by atrophic changes that occur over a 15 to 20 year span. After another 15 or 20 years, the atrophy becomes severe enough that one can make a pathologic diagnosis of gastric atrophy. Eradication of *C. pylori* infection (McNulty, et al., 1986) results in resolution of the chronic, type B gastritis. Both bismuth and amoxicillin eradicate the organism and effect a cure of the gastritis.

The situation is less clear in the case of peptic ulcer because inoculation experiments have failed to demonstrate the development of ulcers as a result of infection with *C. pylori* as opposed to the consistent appearance of acute, superficial gastritis that matures into a characteristic, chronic gastritis. Clearly, physicians should keep track of the literature that is clarifying the importance of *C. pylori* infections of gastric mucosa because there may result important diagnostic and therapeutic procedures that are noninvasive and effective for one or more of these diseases.

Pernicious anemia is considered to be a disease of old age. It is associated with diffuse, atrophic, fundic gland gastritis and with hypo- or achlorhydria, but these conditions are also common in older people without pernicious anemia. This same, confusing overlap is true of parietal cell antibodies in older patients with or without pernicious anemia. About 20 per cent of normal, old people have parietal alloantibodies in their serum—only a few of those with alloantibodies have pernicious anemia. The question of whether these patients and those with gastritis after gastric resection for ulcers should undergo endoscopic survey in search of early cancer has been raised by some investigators who have found in their patient population an increased incidence of gastric cancer. Not everyone agrees with these findings, and some who do are unsure of the utility of searching for early cancer by means of frequent, screening endoscopy in this population. Practical considerations, coupled with lack of proof that such expensive management helps, suggest that one remain circumspect about the problem.

Of the "specific" kinds of gastritis—Ménétrier's, eosinophilic, granulomatous, parasitic, infectious, and irradiation-induced—only the last may have a predilection for older patients because they are more likely to have received irradiation treatment for neoplasm or ulcer. All these kinds of gastritis occur in the aged, however, and should not be excluded from consideration during the construction of a differential diagnosis of a peculiar-looking stomach.

MALIGNANCIES

A study of 296 patients with malignancies of the stomach (Adashek, et al., 1979) indicates that adenocarcinomas and lymphomas occur from the third to the tenth decade; the average age is about 65 for both diseases. Leiomyosarcomas were found in persons of older mean age, but there were only two of these rare cancers in the series. Adenocarcinoma of the stomach has a multifaceted etiology that includes heredity, diet, hypo- or achlorhydria, and exposure to nitroso- compounds and other carcinogens. The incidence in the United States has dropped considerably during this century. Many epidemiologists attribute this reduction to the use of refrigeration to preserve meat instead of smoking it or using other traditional methods.

PEPTIC ULCER

This common disease is said to manifest itself entirely differently when encountered in the elderly than it does in younger patients. Because the population greater than 65 years of age is increasing, this assertion suggests that we must adjust our thinking about the disease. The incidence of ulcers in older women approaches that in older men, and a gastric site is more common in both (Coggon, et al., 1981). It appears that alcohol, smoking, and caffeine are insignificant causative agents in the elderly; however, associated disease, stress, and the use of many drugs play an important part. Aspirin and other anti-inflammatory drugs are commonly used for aches and pains by the elderly, and a small percentage of them suffer complications from the use of these drugs. Of patients older than 65 years, 40 per cent admitted for bleeding and 30 per cent admitted for perforation were taking anti-inflammatory drugs (Watson, 1985).

Vague manifestations, intractability, and reduced rate of recurrence seem to be the hallmarks of the ulcer syndrome in older patients. The pain may not have its usual rhythmicity and relief by antacid. It may be overshadowed by anorexia and weight loss, or it may be absent altogether, the ulcer having been announced by the development of a major complication such as hemorrhage or perforation. Pain was absent in 35 per cent of older patients in one series as opposed to its absence in a mere 8 per cent of a group of young individuals (Clinch, et al., 1984). Furthermore, the clinical presentation may be dominated by systemic symptoms such as the effect of anemia on the cardiovascular system. Thus, dyspnea may be a symptom that finds its ultimate explanation in an ulcer that has leaked blood until the resultant anemia has caused heart failure.

Bleeding is much more severe in the elderly; they require more blood (4.5 versus 2.6 units), and they bleed more often (40 per cent versus 18 per cent). When hemorrhage is caused by gastric ulcer, it has a mortality that is double that of a bleeding duodenal ulcer (Permutt & Cello, 1982). One third of patients older than 70 years do not survive hemorrhage from a gastric ulcer. Half of the bleeding episodes were unheralded by previous ulcer symptoms. Also, hemorrhage from gastric ulcers tended to recur during hospitalization.

Management of such patients requires an urgent, more aggressive approach than is required for the young (Levrat, et al., 1966). The fragile cardiovascular system, the tendency of the bleeding to recur and to be severe, and the debility caused by treatment all argue for an accurate, timely diagnosis and for aggressive attempts to stop the hemorrhage.

Endoscopic evaluation, although not proven to affect mortality, is logical to establish gastric location with its high mortality and frequent requirement for surgical treatment, to look for a visible vessel that predicts rebleeding, and to permit treatment of those cases amenable to endoscopic, therapeutic measures. The visible vessel concept has been controversial, but I believe it is a useful guide. Of 826 patients examined by upper gastrointestinal endoscopy because of bleeding, 402 were found to have peptic ulcers. Of the 329 ulcer craters that could be examined adequately, 156 contained within them a visible vessel. When assigned to a standard, noninvasive treatment, 58 per cent of this group rebled compared with only 6 per cent of the group without a visible vessel (Swain, et al., 1986). These findings indicate that the visible vessel is an identifier of a group of patients who should be watched very closely!

Rebleeding is often an indication for surgical intervention so one attempts to identify the subset of patients in whom this will occur. Large initial hemorrhage, hematemesis preceding admission to the hospital, chronic gastric ulcer, and esophageal varices are associated with recurrent hemorrhage (MacLeod & Mills, 1982). A hemorrhage-free state for 48 hours after admission suggests that rebleeding will not occur. Old age probably correlates with rehemorrhage, but disagreement is found in the literature (Northfield, 1971). In one series of 389 patients, 18 per cent of those less than 60 years of age suffered recurrent hemorrhage, whereas 34 per cent of those greater than 60 years of age rebled. Arteriosclerotic blood vessels of the stomach are not the cause of this problem because arteriosclerosis is not found in these small vessels when they are examined histologically.

The therapeutic effect of drugs for the treatment of hemorrhage has not been settled (Hoare, et al., 1979). Patients older than 45 years who were hospitalized for significant gastrointestinal hemorrhage were treated with placebo (N = 32) or cimetidine (N = 34) in a dosage of 200 mg every four hours for 48 hours, followed by 400 mg four times a day for one week. Transfusion requirements of the two groups were equal. Eight treated and 13 control patients continued to bleed. Emergency operations for bleeding were required in three and four instances, respectively.

Special consideration should be given to the dosage and the side effects of medicines used to treat the elderly. A study by Greene and colleagues (1985) of healthy volunteers given rantidine twice daily for seven doses indicated that those who were older than 50 years exhibited higher plasma concentrations and longer half-lives than younger subjects. No clinical effects were attributed to these pharmacological differences, but one should be aware of the possibility of toxicity and of exaggerated effects of other drugs, particularly when H_2 blockers are used to treat hemorrhage in older patients.

If one combines the results of ten studies of cimetidine versus placebo in gastrointestinal hemorrhage (Falk, et al., 1985), one sees no clear benefit of treatment with the drug. Of a total of 527 patients treated and 520 control subjects, rebleeding occurred 96 versus 107 times, surgical treatment 85 versus 92 times, and death 29 versus 36 times, respectively. If the gastric ulcer subgroups were isolated, there was a trend toward treatment benefit with respect to rebleeding and reduced need for surgical intervention. For practical purposes, it seems logical to employ H_2 blockade in the management of bleeding ulcers, especially when they are gastric and when drug interactions are unlikely.

Sucralfate has been compared with cimetidine for efficacy in the treatment of bleeding peptic ulcers. There was no difference in a small group of patients; the question of whether or not either is an improvement over placebo was not answered. At least sucralfate caused no side effects (Goldfarb & Czaja, 1985).

Investigators continue to search for a drug that is clearly effective in the treatment of gastrointestinal hemorrhage, particularly in the elderly. Topical prostaglandin E_2 did not control hemorrhage in one study (Levine, et al., 1985), but it accelerated healing as judged by endoscopic criteria. Somatostatin (Magnusson, et al., 1985), which is a potent inhibitor of gastric secretion of acid, pepsin, and intrinsic factor as well as of splanchnic blood flow, reduced the number of operations in a treated group versus a group given placebo (1 versus 5) but did not reduce the mortality or the incidence of rebleeding. If further work confirms that somatostatin reduces the need for surgical treatment of such patients, the drug will become part of our standard regimen.

Laser therapy has also been used in an attempt to reduce mortality or the need for surgical treatment of upper gastrointestinal hemorrhage due to ulcer. In a community hospital study of 71 patients bleeding from the gastrointestinal tract, Overholt (1985) was able to stop hemorrhage in 79 per cent of the gastric ulcer patients. Five of these required a second laser treatment, and six patients required a surgical procedure. One patient died because of laser-induced hemorrhage. These results and others like them are encouraging but are a long way from satisfactory when one recalls that about 80 per cent of the gastrointestinal hemorrhage stops promptly, and that the 8 to 10 per cent mortality rate seen a half a century ago persists. Similar results are reported by those who use other methods of coagulating vessels such as heater probes or bicap.

Ultimately, there is a group of patients with such persistent or severe hemorrhage that surgical measures must be employed to save their lives. There are risks—some from the nature of the clinical condition, some from errors in judgment, some from the fact that sick, old people are subject to a higher incidence of mortality following surgery. The fact that a study comparing surgical experience in 1982 with that in 1972 showed no difference in mortality or average age (Kim, et al., 1985), but a reduction of unidentified bleeding sites from 25 to 0 per cent over a decade, suggests that the risk of dying is patient-driven. The higher incidence of gastritis in the 1982 study, particularly in those who were not admitted for gastrointestinal hemorrhage, seems to bear this out.

Certainly if surgical mortality is to be reduced, one must avoid emergency operations. At the Peter Bent Brigham Hospital in 1964 (Brooks & Eraklis, 1964), the mortality rate for elective subtotal gastrectomy was 0.4 per cent as opposed to a 21 per cent mortality rate when the operation was done as an emergency for gastrointestinal hemorrhage. The patients with the higher mortality rate were often older than the others, and their mortality was caused by failure of a major organ system, usually the lungs or the heart (Allan & Dykes, 1976).

A word is in order about the treatment of ulcers after the bleeding stops. Alternatives to standard antacid treatment have been described in the section on the treatment of the bleeding gastric ulcer. Others are also being tried. They include omeprazole, a hydrogen potassium ATPase inhibitor, which is fast and very effective (Bardhan, et al., 1986). Its effect on recurrence is not well known. Milk, when given in the amount usually recommended in the past, actually increases acid secretion and decreases healing percentage. It is wise to avoid milk in the treatment of older people (Kumar, et al., 1986). Furthermore, one should be cautious about the amount of H_2 blocker one uses in the elderly. The amount of reduction of acid required for successful ulcer treatment may be less than traditionally believed. If this is true, one could reduce the dose of drug, whether it be H_2 inhibitor, antacid, or omeprazole, and have a consequent reduction in the risk of side effects. This is a very important benefit in the older age population.

OTHER CAUSES OF HEMORRHAGE

In the consideration of bleeding ulcer, one should also be aware of some less mundane causes of hemorrhage even if an ulcer is present. Older patients frequently have hiatus hernias, and all manner of symptoms have been unwisely attributed to them. The Mayo group has found a possible association, however, with linear gastric erosion (Cameron & Higgins, 1986). Located only in the body of the stomach near the constriction caused by the diaphragm, these linear, frequently multiple, erosions are aligned with the axis of a gastric fold, which is usually swollen and red. They appear intermittently and are not related to aspirin use. Discovery of such lesions can afford diagnostic refuge during the management of puzzling instances of iron deficiency anemia.

The older patient is known to be prone to angiodysplasia of the cecum, but these lesions also occur in the stomach and duodenum (Gunnlaugsson, 1985). Twenty-five angiodysplastic lesions were found in a series of 1030 gastroscopies. The patients had no evidence of Osler-Weber-Rendu disease, but they sometimes had valvular heart disease. The lesions were occasionally found in other parts of the gut as well (Clouse, et al., 1985).

When gastrointestinal bleeding is massive, one considers aortoenteric fistula. This is unfortunate because in a study of 13 patients with this problem, none were in shock and only one fainted. Failure to consider this diagnosis when the bleeding is not severe is one reason for the mortality of 60 to 70 per cent (O'Donnell, et al., 1985). If a patient with an aortic graft has a gastrointestinal hemorrhage with a negative endoscopy, consider the diagnosis. The most frequent location of the fistula is in the third or fourth part of the duodenum.

Perforation

Perforation is the second ranking complication of peptic ulcer. Gastric perforations are more dangerous than the more common duodenal ones. In patients older than 75 years, the mortality rate is almost 50 per cent (Steinheber, 1985). The major cause of this sad state of affairs is failure to reach an early diagnosis; a delay of 24 hours is common (25 per cent). This underestimate of the gravity of the abdominal event is caused by minimal physical findings, lack of history of an ulcer, and by major signs that other organs are failing, thus directing the attention of the physician away from the ultimate cause of the trouble, a perforated ulcer. Adding to the confusion is the frequent presence of other serious, chronic diseases (Ng & Batey, 1986).

One important clue to perforated ulcer can be the history of the use of nonsteroidal anti-inflammatory drugs. Of 78 patients who died of perforated or bleeding ulcer (44 died either at home or in the emergency unit before they could be operated on), sixty-one (78 per cent) were taking nonsteroidal anti-inflammatory drugs versus 8 per cent of the matched controls admitted for other emergency conditions. There is also a significant correlation ($P < 0.001$) between the annual number of perforated peptic ulcers in patients older than 65 who take nonsteroidal anti-inflammatory drugs and the annual number of prescriptions for these drugs issued in the region being studied.

Although most elderly patients with a perforated ulcer complain of abdominal distress, fully one in six describe minimal abdominal pain, and most of them have had pain longer than six hours before they seek medical care—a very unusual finding in younger patients with a perforated ulcer. Occasionally, there are no findings when the abdominal examination is conducted (Kane, et al., 1981). The problem is further complicated by the fact that free air is so often absent in roentgenograms (40 per cent in a series of 32 patients greater than 60 years of age).

The problem seems particularly difficult for an internist because most surgical patients have severe abdominal pain, whereas only 3 out of 14 medical patients complain of that symptom (Coleman & Denham, 1980). Instead, they report general malaise, nausea, vomiting, hematemesis, or melena, which is why they are sent to an internist. Moreover, 10 out of 14 medical patients were confused or obtunded as opposed to none of 24 surgical patients. The resultant inaccurate or absent histories will clearly cause great difficulty.

MISCELLANEOUS EFFECTS OF GASTRECTOMY

Standard treatment protocols have required that patients who have had gastrectomies should have surveillance for "stump cancer" (Schuman, 1986). The disease is believed to increase with time, occurring 20 years postgastrectomy. Modern recommendations suggest a screening endoscopy the twentieth year after the gastrectomy and every five years thereafter. If biopsies indicate the presence of dysplasia, adenoma, or metaplasia, the intervals should be decreased to two or three years. Highly selective vagotomy patients are not at increased risk; standard vagotomy patients are. The issue is still in doubt, however, so these recommendations may be changed at any time when data are more compelling.

Finally, one should be aware that significant bone disease is frequent after gastric surgery (Klein, et al., 1987). It becomes manifest after ten years and can be associated with vertebral fractures in as many as three out of four patients. Osteomalacia and osteoporosis are both present in many instances. Symptoms may be absent or they may be debilitating. If such a problem is burdensome for a healthy person, it can be a disaster for a weak, older patient.

THERAPEUTIC MISADVENTURES

Drug Therapy

Because cancer is a degenerative disease seen most often in older people, one finds complications of cancer treatment in them. A particularly fascinating side effect of treatment is gastroduodenal mucosal injury when chemotherapeutic agents are infused into the hepatic artery for the purpose of treating hepatic metastases (Mavligit, et al., 1987). Anatomical vascular aberrations cause the drug to perfuse parts of the stomach 30 to 40 per cent of the time, leading to a dyspeptic syndrome with inflammation of the mucosa or the development of an ulcer. Attempts to avoid this by the use of H_2 blockade or prostaglandin E_1 analogs have failed.

Therapeutic Endoscopy

When degenerative diseases affect the gastrointestinal tract, e.g., dysphagia after stroke, the gastroenterologist is called upon to help because there is an increasing armamentarium available for use in such patients. These invasive treatments and diagnostic techniques have a price—occasional complications.

Bacteremia occurs with endoscopy, but has a low frequency (2 to 6 per cent) for most procedures including colonoscopy and endoscopic retrograde cholangiopancreatography (ERCP). When esophageal dilatation or variceal sclerotherapy is done, however, there is a 30 to 40 per cent incidence of bacteremia. Although both gram-negative and gram-positive organisms are found, the infrequent bacterial endocarditis that occurs after these procedures is usually caused by the gram-positive organisms (Botoman & Surawica, 1986). Prophylaxis is recommended by the American Heart Association, even though proof of effectiveness is weak. Prudence dictates antibiotic prophylaxis for all patients with prosthetic heart valves no matter which endoscopic procedure is employed. A history of endocarditis is another indication. Those who have valvular disease require prophylaxis when esophageal dilatation or variceal sclerotherapy is employed. These recommendations are sensible but empirical. Since the cumulative risk for bacteremia from chewing and related activity is many-fold greater than that for endoscopy, one wonders whether any good is accomplished.

The antibiotic regimens recently recommended call for the use of ampicillin or amoxicillin with gentamycin, amoxicillin alone, or vancomycin and gentamycin when the patient is allergic to penicillin. Two doses are given, one before the procedure and one six to eight hours later.

Intraperitoneal hemorrhage from tearing of the vessels in the gastrosplenic ligament has been reported after a gastroscopy. This rare, therefore easily missed, event requires surgical treatment so it is worth remembering (Pricolo & Cipolleta, 1987).

Pneumoperitoneum after endoscopy is well known (Gottfried, et al., 1986). It also occurs with some frequency (40 percent) after percutaneous endoscopic gastrostomy (PEG). Usually, no treatment is required. A more dangerous complication of PEG is necrotizing fasciitis/myositis. In a case reported by Person and Brower (1986), it took six days for the problem to manifest enough signs to localize it to the gastrostomy site. The inflamed, necrotic tissue was extensively débrided; cultures supported the growth of *Staphylococcus aureus* and Enterobacteriaceae. Tight seal of the skin around the gastrostomy tube may have been a risk factor contributing to this complication.

CONCLUSION

Although the diseases of the stomach encountered in the old patient are largely the same common ailments that afflict the young, their manifestations are often quite different. Dominance of systemic symptoms or manifestations of vital organ failure (kidney, heart, lungs) may cloud the clinical picture, resulting in a delayed or missed diagnosis. This is particularly true of perforated ulcer. Alterations of memory in the aged may render the history, that bulwark of clinical medicine, useless. The presence of multiple diseases also misdirects the attention of the physician in some instances. Nevertheless, the experienced clinician who conducts a thoughtful bedside examination, utilizes the large laboratory armamentarium parsimoniously and wisely, and has a little luck will miss few of these diseases. They are not rare; they are merely surprising in their manifestations.

REFERENCES

Achem-Karam, S.R., et al.: Plasma motilin concentration and interdigestive migrating motor complex in diabetic gastroparesis: Effect of metoclopramide. Gastroenterology 88:492–499, 1985.

Adashek, K., et al.: Cancer of the stomach. Review of consecutive 10 year intervals. Ann Surg 189:6, 1979.

Allan, R., and Dykes, P.: A study of the factors influencing mortality rates from gastrointestinal haemorrhage. Q J Med 45:533–550, 1976.

Bardhan, K.D., et al.: A comparison of two different doses of omeprazole versus ranitidine in treatment of duodenal ulcers. J Clin Gastroenterol 8:408–413, 1986.

Barr, H., et al: Who should have endocarditis prophylaxis for upper gastrointestinal procedures? (letters to the editor). Gastrointest Endosc 32:302–303, 1986.

Botoman, V.A., and Surawica, C.M.: Bacteremia with gastrointestinal endoscopic procedures. Gastrointest Endosc 32:342–345, 1986.

Brooks, J.R., and Eraklis, A.J.: Factors affecting the mortality from peptic ulcer. N Engl J Med 271:803–809, 1964.

Cameron, A.J., and Higgins, J.A.: Linear gastric erosion—A lesion associated with large diaphragmatic hernia and chronic blood loss anemia. Gastroenterology 91:338–342, 1986.

Clinch, D., et al: Absence of abdominal pain in elderly patients with peptic ulcer. Age Aging 13:120–123, 1984.

Clouse, R.E., et al.: Angiodysplasia as a cause of upper gastrointestinal bleeding. Arch Intern Med 145:458–461, 1985.

Coggon, D., et al.: 20 Years of hospital admissions for peptic ulcer in England and Wales. Lancet 1:1302–1304, 1981.

Cole, H.M. (ed.): (Questions & answers) Diagnostic and therapeutic technology assessment (DATTA). JAMA 256:1358–1359, 1986.

Coleman, J.A., and Denham, M.J.: Perforation of peptic ulceration in the elderly. Age Aging 9:257–261, 1980.

Collier, D.S., and Pain, J.A.: Non-steroidal anti-inflammatory drugs and peptic ulcer perforation. Gut 26:359–363, 1985.

Domschke, S., and Domschke, W.: Gastroduodenal damage due to drugs, alcohol and smoking. Clin Gastroenterol 13:405–436, 1984.

Falk, A., et al.: Histamine$_2$ receptor antagonists in gastroduodenal ulcer haemorrhage. Scand J Gastroenterol 20:95–100, 1985.

Geokas, M.C., et al.: The aging gastrointestinal tract, liver, and pancreas. Clin Geriatr Med 1:177–205, 1985.

Goldfarb, J.P., and Czaja, M.J.: A comparison of cimetidine and sucralfate in the treatment of bleeding peptic ulcers. Am J Gastroenterol 80:5–7, 1985.

Gottfried, E.B., et al.: Pneumoperitoneum following percutaneous endoscopic gastrostomy. Gastrointest Endosc 32:397–399, 1986.

Greene, D.S., et al.: The effect of age on ranitidine pharmacokinetics. Gastroenterology 88:1662, 1985.

Greenburg, A.G., et al.: Changing patterns of gastrointestinal bleeding. Arch Surg 120:341–344, 1985.

Gunnlaugsson, O.: Angiodysplasia of the stomach and duodenum. Gastrointest Endosc 31:251–254, 1985.

Hazell, S.L., and Graham, D.Y.: *Campylobacter pylori* in perspective. Pract Gastroenterol 12:11–21, 1988.

Hoare, A.M., et al.: Cimetidine in bleeding peptic ulcer. Lancet, 2:671–673, 1979.

Hogan, R. B., et al.: Percutaneous endoscopic gastrostomy—to push or pull. Gastrointest Endosc 32:253–258, 1986.

Holt, P.R.: What to feed the patient with an aging GI tract. Pract Gastroenterol 11:17–18, 1987.

Kane, E., et al.: Perforated peptic ulcer in the elderly. J Am Geriatr Soc 24:224–227, 1981.

Kim, B., et al.: Risks of surgery for upper gastrointestinal hemorrhage: 1972 versus 1982. Am J Surg 149:474–476, 1985.

Klein, K.B., et al.: Metabolic bone disease in asymptomatic men after partial gastrectomy with Billroth II anastomosis. Gastroenterology 92:608–615, 1987.

Kumar, N., et al.: Effect of milk on patients with duodenal ulcers. Br Med J 293:666, 1986.

Kurata, J.H., et al.: Sex differences in peptic ulcer disease. Gastroenterology 88:96–100, 1985.

Kurata, J.H., et al.: A reappraisal of time trends in ulcer disease: Factors related to changes in ulcer hospitalization and mortality rates. Am J Public Health 73:1066–1072, 1983.

Levine, B.A., et al.: Topical prostaglandin E_2 in the treatment of acute upper gastrointestinal tract hemorrhage. Arch Surg 120:600–604, 1985.

Levrat, M., et al.: Peptic ulcer in patients over 60. Experience in 287 cases. Am J Dig Dis 11:279–285, 1966.

Lipschitz, D.A. (Moderator), et al.: Conference—Cancer in the elderly: Basic science and clinical aspects. Ann Intern Med 102:218–228, 1985.

MacLeod, I.A., and Mills, P.R.: Factors identifying the probability of further haemorrhage after acute upper gastrointestinal haemorrhage. Br J Surg 69:256–258, 1982.

Magnusson, I., et al.: Randomised double blind trial of somatostatin in the treatment of massive upper gastrointestinal haemorrhage. Gut 26:221–226, 1985.

Mavligit, G.M., et al.: Gastroduodenal mucosal injury during hepatic arterial infusion of chemotherapeutic agents. Gastroenterology 92:566–569, 1987.

McManus, J.P.: Differing incidence and long latency of malignancy after gastric surgery. Gastroenterology 92:1309–1310, 1986.

McManus, J.P.: How much less acid and no ulcer? Gastroenterology 90:2027–2028, 1986.

McNulty, C.A.M., et al.: *Campylobacter pylorielis* and acid induced gastric metaplasia: Investigator blind, placebo controlled trial of bismuth salicylate and erythromycin ethylsuccinate. Br Med J 293:645–649, 1986.

Murakami, M., et al.: Pathogenesis and pathophysiology of chronic gastric ulcer in elderly patients. Gastroenterology 88:1512, 1985.

Narayanan, M., and Steinheber, F.U.: The changing face of peptic ulcer in the elderly. Med Clin North Am 60:1159–1172, 1976.

Ng, J., and Batey, R.: Letters to the Editor. Lancet 1:972, 1986.

Northfield, T.C.: Factors predisposing to recurrent haemorrhage after acute gastrointestinal bleeding. Br Med J 1:26–28, 1971.

O'Donnell, T.F., Jr., et al.: Improvements in the diagnosis and management of aortoenteric fistula. Am J Surg 149:481–486, 1985.

Overholt, B.F.: Laser treatment of upper gastrointestinal hemorrhage. Am J Gastroenterol 80:721–726, 1985.

Permutt, R.P., and Cello, J.P.: Duodenal ulcer disease in the hospitalized elderly patient. Dig Dis Sci 27:1–6, 1982.

Person, J.L., and Brower, R.A.: Necrotizing fasciitis/myositis following percutaneous endoscopic gastrostomy. Gastrointest Endosc 32:309, 1986.

Pricolo, R., and Cipolletta, L.: Intraperitoneal hemorrhage following upper gastrointestinal endoscopy. Gastrointest Endosc 33:53–54, 1987.

Schuman, B.M.: Endoscopic surveillance for cancer of the gastric stump. Gastrointest Endosc 32:117–118, 1986.

Sleisenger, M.H., and Fordtran, J.S.: Gastrointestinal Disease: Pathophysiology, Diagnosis, Management. 3rd ed. Philadelphia, W.B. Saunders Company, 1983.

Somerville, K., et al.: Non-steroidal anti-inflammatory drugs and bleeding peptic ulcer. Lancet 1:462–464, 1986.

Steinheber, F.U.: Ageing and the stomach. Clin Gastroenterol 14:657–688, 1985.

Sterup, K., and Mosbech, J.: Trends in the mortality from peptic ulcer in Denmark. Scand J Gastroenterol 8:49–53, 1972.

Swain, C.P., et al.: Nature of the bleeding vessel in recurrently bleeding gastric ulcers. Gastroenterology 90:595–608, 1986.

Wara, P.: Endoscopic prediction of major rebleeding—A prospective study of stigmata of hemorrhage in bleeding ulcer. Gastroenterology 88:1209–1214, 1985.

Warren, J.R., and Marshall, B.J.: Unidentified curved bacillin on gastric epithelium in active chronic gastritis. Lancet 1:1273–1275, 1983.

Watson, R.J., et al: Duodenal ulcer disease in the elderly: A retrospective study. Age Aging 14:225–229, 1985.

Chapter 3
SMALL INTESTINE
William A. Sodeman, Jr.

The small intestine is no less susceptible to the aging process than any other component of the digestive tract. However, changes related to aging of the intestine, and in particular disease as a direct consequence of aging, have been extraordinarily difficult to document in humans. A number of diseases involving the small intestine increase in frequency in the elderly, but they are not related directly to the aging process in the intestine. The small intestine is also secondarily involved in aging processes that involve the vascular system.

AGE-RELATED CHANGES IN THE SMALL INTESTINE

Morphology

Aging brings gross and microscopic structural changes in the small intestine. Flattening of villi and increased numbers of leaf-shaped villi have been reported in the elderly (Webster & Leeming, 1975). These changes are not known to be of clinical significance.

There is a wealth of investigation involving animal observations that describes small intestinal changes with aging at the cellular level, including cell turnover rates and changes in the diffusion barrier. It is likely that some similar changes also occur in humans, but none have been demonstrated convincingly (Holt, 1985).

Jejunal Diverticula

Acquired jejunal diverticula may occur in patients with collagen-vascular diseases at any age. Congenital diverticula occur but not with the frequency of duodenal diverticulum or Meckel's diverticulum. Otherwise, simple jejunal diverticulosis seems to be a problem in patients over age 50. These are false diverticula that occur on the mesenteric border at the points of penetration of nutrient arteries through the muscular wall of the intestine. This suggests etiologically the occurrence of increased intralumenal pressure in functionally closed loops of jejunum, with eventual herniation of the mucosa through these weak points in the small intestinal wall. It is not clear whether the pathophysiology involves abnormal motility as a result of aging or simply an age-related increase in the frequency of development of functionally closed loops under high intralumenal pressure.

Clinically these diverticula are usually silent. They can, of course, be susceptible to any of the complications of diverticula, i.e., obstruction, bleeding, inflammation, perforation, enterolith formation, adhesion formation, and, if large or massed, bacterial overgrowth. Bacterial overgrowth will be discussed later in this chapter. A barium contrast x-ray, particularly with delayed films (Fig. 3–1), is most likely to make the diagnosis in the absence of complication. Treatment is limited to that necessary to respond to complications (Spiro, 1983).

Motility

A single study (Anuras & Sutherland, 1984) showed no abnormal contractions but just a slight decrease in their frequency, with the

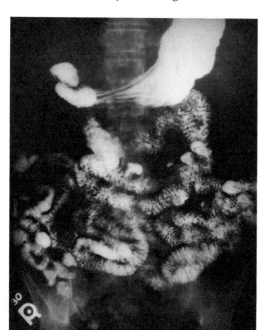

Figure 3–1. This barium contrast x-ray with 30 minutes delay shows multiple jejunal diverticula.

conclusion that an older small intestine is simply somewhat less active. The interdigestive motor complex, often called the intestinal house-keeper, remains intact in the aged.

Absorption

Aging produces gross changes in the absorption of nutrients, but many mechanisms (including gastric atrophy and age-related changes in pancreatic exocrine function) may be contributors. The contribution of the small intestine to this malabsorption has proven deceptively difficult to document. Impairment in absorption of carbohydrates, fats, and proteins has been demonstrated in a number of animal models of the aging process, but technical difficulties have made it difficult to confirm in humans. A carefully done study of d-xylose absorption which took into account alterations in renal function did demonstrate a defect in absorption in patients over 63, but the defect was minor (Webster & Leeming, 1975). Feibusch and Holt (1979) using breath hydrogen assay demonstrated an impairment in mixed carbohydrate absorption in one third of patients over age 65.

Absorption of fat and protein is often impaired, but it is not clear that the small intestine's contribution to the pathophysiology of the malabsorption is significant. With the exception of calcium there is little evidence that the small intestine plays a role in the deficiency of minerals or vitamins in the elderly. A number of studies summarized by Holt (1985) show a decrease in calcium absorption in the elderly. The mechanism is in dispute, but it is of clinical significance that absorption is normalized with the administration of vitamin D (calcif-erol). While the net result of these changes in absorption is not clinically significant in a healthy individual, these changes do narrow the reserve in the elderly, who then become susceptible to small deficiencies in nutrition.

Summary

Despite all the gaps in our understanding of the age-related changes in motility and absorption in the small intestine, there are some useful clinical observations. Jejunal *diverticulosis* does occur with aging. Jejunal *diverticulitis*, although it is uncommon, is a diagnostic dilemma as it occurs in an area anatomically isolated from application of most of the newer diagnostic techniques.

The absorptive reserve of the small intestine is large. Nature repeatedly forces the trauma surgeon to demonstrate this absorptive reserve by resection of varying lengths of damaged small intestine. Although changes in absorption as a result of aging are small individually, collectively they are additive and, in conjunction with other digestive or metabolic abnormalities or nutritional deficiency, may become clinically evident. Schneider and coworkers (1986) emphasize that the physiological changes associated with aging will affect the need for nutrients, vitamins, and minerals. As a positive feature, because multiple mechanisms are at work, the physician often has several different opportunities to try to restore nutritional balance. Small supplements or successful treatment involving a minor absorptive pathway may rescue a fragile balance even in the face of irreversible pathological change of major absorptive routes.

DISEASES WITH INCREASED FREQUENCY IN THE AGED

Gluten-Sensitive Enteropathy (Celiac Disease, Nontropical Sprue)

A recent review has suggested that at least one quarter of the cases of gluten-sensitive enteropathy will first appear after age 70 (Swinson & Levi, 1980). The sensitivity to gluten and the underlying pathological appearance of the intestinal mucosa are similar at any age. However, the clinical presentation in the elderly may be strikingly different. The disease is often masked, without the overt signs of malabsorption, anemia, and the calcium deficiency common in younger age groups. These traditional elements of the disease along with bleeding tendency, neuropathy, and edema share many more frequent etiologies in the elderly and thus the clinical problem is largely one of remembering to include gluten-sensitive enteropathy in the differential diagnosis and to be willing to move to small bowel biopsy when evidence for more common etiologies is lacking. Small bowel biopsy remains the method for a diagnosis, which is then corroborated by response to gluten exclusion.

Treatment with gluten exclusion is as effective in the elderly as it is in the young. The restrictive nature of the diet does require rigorous follow-up to ensure not only compliance with gluten exclusion but also the continued adequacy of overall nutrition. Two complications of gluten-sensitive enteropathy seem more frequent in the elderly. Multiple small intestinal ulcers have been observed to occur even when the patient is in remission of a gluten-free diet. Approximately one fifth of the cases are patients over age 60. Diarrhea and weight loss occur but with the addition of abdominal pain and fever. Often the first signs of ulceration are the complications of hemorrhage, perforation, and/or obstruction. Diagnosis is difficult; neither x-ray nor endoscopy have much to offer. Surgical intervention seems to offer the best hope for survival in the face of complications (Baer, et al., 1980).

Increase in the frequency of malignancy is a well-identified complication of gluten-sensitive enteropathy. Frequency of occurrence of tumor increases with the age of the patient and the duration of disease. Both carcinomas and lymphomas occur. Small intestinal lymphomas are most frequent. An unexpected response to gluten exclusion, with either a failure to respond in newly diagnosed patients or a relapse in an established patient, should prompt the addition of malignancy to the differential diagnosis (Holmes, et al., 1976).

Diabetic Autonomic Neuropathy

Diabetic Diarrhea

Among the complications of longstanding diabetes is visceral neuropathy. This results in diarrhea and somewhat less frequently in a pseudo-obstruction syndrome. Visceral neuropathy occurs in patients with insulin-dependent diabetes and is a late complication. Usually there is an associated peripheral neuropathy. The diarrhea is watery and may occur both day and night. The nocturnal diarrhea receives most attention because of the frequent association with fecal incontinence, which is emotionally and socially crippling to the elderly patient. The course is often remittent, although the causes of exacerbation and remission are unknown. At least four pathophysiological mechanisms are postulated—steatorrhea, bacterial overgrowth, altered motility (autonomic neuropathy), and altered fluid and electrolyte absorption— and, in truth, all may play a role. In any given patient one may predominate, and with patience and systematic therapeutic trial, there are opportunities to offer symptomatic control.

Steatorrhea

Mild steatorrhea is a common finding in diabetics. The levels of malabsorbed fat would not burden a normal bowel but may be important in a diseased intestine. Steatorrhea would be seen to be additive to diabetic diarrhea of other etiologies (Goyal & Spiro, 1971). In management it seems reasonable to respect limits on dietary fat intake at least to the extent that the dietary control of the diabetes will permit. The use of medium chain triglycerides may also be helpful in promoting fat and calorie absorption. Although the incremental decrease in diarrhea may be small, it need not be clinically insignificant.

Bacterial Overgrowth

Radiological studies demonstrate motility abnormalities with dilated loops of intestine in some patients with visceral neuropathy. This is a setting compatible with bacterial overgrowth. Clinically only a limited number of these patients will improve with antibiotic therapy, probably a reflection of the multiple etiologies of diabetic diarrhea (King & Toskes, 1979). The use of cholestyramine to bind bile salts deconjugated by bacteria has also had limited success.

Visceral Neuropathy

The visceral neuropathy itself may alter motility mechanisms, with a resulting low resistance to aboral intestinal transit. However, it is admitted that this mechanism has yet to be consistently demonstrated (Whalen, et al., 1969). The use of diphenoxylate HCl or loperamide HCl is the mainstay of symptomatic control, particularly of nocturnal diarrhea. It is not clear whether the benefit is an effect on the small or large intestine. Nonabsorbable fiber has also been a useful adjunct in the management of these patients. It acts to convert the semifluid stool to semisolid and offers a little more resistance to uncontrolled transit.

Fluid and Electrolyte Absorption

Recently attention has focused on impaired fluid and electrolyte absorption in both the ileum and the colon, with the defect reversible by the activation of alpha-2 adrenergic receptors. Loss of adrenergic innervation would be the mechanism. In control of the diarrhea, clonidine, an alpha-2 adrenergic agonist, has been used with success in a few patients. Too few patients have been reported to provide guidelines for the safe and effective use of the drug, but it does hold great promise for medical therapy of this difficult problem (Fedorak, et al., 1985).

Pseudo-obstruction

The syndrome of chronic intermittent intestinal pseudo-obstruction also occurs with longstanding insulin-dependent diabetes, but it is not very common. Although autonomic neuropathy is invoked as the cause, the mechanism is not clear. The treatment of acute attacks of obstruction rests with maintenance of fluid and electrolyte balance. The exclusion of other life-threatening causes of obstruction occupies most of one's clinical attention (Anuras, et al., 1978). Constipation is a very common complaint in diabetics, but unlike the diarrhea, it can be comfortably ignored by both patient and physician. Unfortunately, inattention leads to impaction and its complicated management (see Chapter 5).

Syndromes of Bacterial Overgrowth (Stasis, Blind Loop Syndrome)

Bacterial overgrowth gives every evidence of being a real sleeper as a cause of disability among the elderly. It occurs in a number of settings in which an anatomical alteration that permits stasis has been identified. It also has been associated with a number of enteric and systemic problems that result in impaired motility in the small intestine. Recently there has been discussion of impairment of normal defense mechanisms as pathophysiological mechanisms, particularly loss or impairment of the barrier that gastric acid offers against entrance of viable microorganisms into the small intestine and the failure to produce or secrete enteric antibodies (Simon & Gorbach, 1984). Table 3–1 outlines the range of etiologies. Many of these possible etiological mechanisms accumulate in the aging population (King & Toskes, 1979). In addition, there have been three reports concerning the occurrence of bacterial overgrowth in elderly patients without anatomical or other explanations for the phenomenon (Roberts, et al., 1977; McEvoy, et al., 1983; Holt, 1985). In those patients in whom the mechanism involves disturbed motility with stasis rather than blind loop with stasis, such as fistulae-connected recirculation loops, the essential missing function is postulated to be absence or interference with the interdigestive myoelectric complex (often called the intestinal housekeeper). This complex generates a contraction that literally sweeps down the intestine from pylorus to cecum, cleaning and emptying the lumen of secretions, chyme, and bacteria. There is one report of abnormality of this complex in patients with bacterial overgrowth but as yet no report of the frequency of the abnormality in the elderly (VanTrappen, et al., 1977).

Bacterial Nutrient Interactions

Bacterial overgrowth in the small intestine is associated with the development of a malabsorption syndrome. Three features seem to be

TABLE 3–1. Mechanisms of Bacterial Overgrowth

Enhanced Access of Bacteria to the Small Intestine
Achlorhydria
Postgastrectomy +/− vagotomy
Atrophic gastritis
Secondary to gastric antisecretory therapy
Morphological Changes Permitting Stasis in the Small Intestine
Congenital small intestinal diverticula (most frequently duodenal)
Acquired small intestinal diverticula (most frequently jejunal)
Partial small bowel obstruction
Gastrocolic fistula
Ileocolic fistula
Enteroenteric fistula (recirculating small intestinal loop)
Surgical sequelae
Afferent loop of a Billroth II resection
Surgically constructed blind loop (particularly self-filling loops)
Recirculating loop secondary to a side-to-side anastomosis
Resection of the ileocecal valve
Functional Abnormalities in the Small Intestine
Scleroderma
Enteric autonomic neuropathy
Impairment of the interdigestive motor complex

involved as mechanisms. Bacterial consumption of a nutrient is a minor but occasionally significant feature. Binding of B_{12} by aerobic and anaerobic bacteria can effectively compete with intrinsic factor and render the B_{12} unavailable for absorption. Bacteria are capable of producing as well as binding and consuming nutrients. Folic acid is a bacterial product, and increased serum levels occur in the presence of bacterial overgrowth. There is a suggestion that vitamin K may also be a bacterial product (King & Toskes, 1979).

Bile Salt Deconjugation

A second mechanism for the malabsorption involves bacterial metabolism of conjugated bile salts, with the resultant conjugated bile salt deficiency impairing lipid absorption. The deconjugated bile salts may also play a direct role in the development of diarrhea. The level at which the bacteria reside in the intestine affects bacterial access to conjugated bile salts and thus the relative importance of this mechanism to the malabsorptive process (King & Toskes, 1979; Simon & Gorbach, 1984).

Cellular Damage

The third mechanism involved in the development of malabsorption is direct damage to the enterocyte and to the integrity of mucosal function. The differential diagnosis of partial villous atrophy now includes bacterial overgrowth. Decrease or loss of the enzyme activities associated with enterocyte function is described. Protein-losing and fat-losing enteropathies have also been described. The damage does not appear to represent infection of the mucosa but rather direct and/or toxic effects of the bacteria and metabolic products of bacterial action on the mucosal epithelial cell. Whatever the mechanism, the lesions appear to be reversible with elimination of bacterial overgrowth (King & Toskes, 1979). Changes in the brush border enzyme of dogs with bacterial overgrowth have been described (Batt, et al., 1984).

Clinical Diagnosis

The spectrum of clinical presentation of patients with bacterial overgrowth is large and varied. A single feature such as a macrocytic anemia may dominate the clinical presentation, or there may be severe malnutrition with multiple nutritional defects. Thus, bacterial overgrowth must be included in the differential diagnosis even when the first diagnostic choice is gastric atrophy or colon cancer. Failure to confirm the likely diagnosis in an elderly patient presenting with any sort of malnutrition should prompt consideration of bacterial overgrowth syndrome. Perhaps the most difficult diagnosis is in the patient who presents with the geriatric equivalent of failure to thrive but without nutritional or anatomical explanation for the malnutrition. As mentioned in the beginning of this section, there have been several reports of apparent bacterial overgrowth in the absence of predisposing cause all described in elderly patients—a diagnostic dilemma best resolved by a breath test rather than a therapeutic trial of antibiotics.

Laboratory Diagnosis

Confirmation of the diagnosis can be done with a high degree of accuracy by demonstrating the presence of bacterial flora in the small intestine. Overgrowth is defined as the presence of greater than 10^5 organisms per ml of aspirate. Anaerobic bacteria are more likely than aerobic flora to be the culprits. Proper culture requires the intubation of the small intestine, then anaerobic aspiration of intestinal contents with rapid transfer to an anaerobic culture system for a quantitative culture. The invasive part of the test—the intubation—is technically not difficult but can be time consuming and is uncomfortable for the patient. Repeat culture, sometimes necessary in follow-up, may be particularly trying to the elderly patient. The real problem in obtaining an accurate quantitative culture rests with the isolation of anaerobes, which does require properly equipped laboratory facilities. In many hospitals, the necessary laboratory resources are simply not available.

Indirect Assays

Because of the difficulties in isolating the flora, a number of indirect assays for the presence of bacterial overgrowth have been tried. All are useful; none has proven ideal. Testing the aspirate for the presence of deconjugated bile acids is a research procedure. Assay of 24-hour urine collections for the presence of indican has been used as an indirect test for bacterial overgrowth. Indican is the final product of intralumenal, bacterial degradation of tryptophan. Unfortunately, urinary levels do not discriminate between small intestinal and colonic flora, and thus the sensitivity of the test is limited.

At the present time most attention centers on breath analysis— analysis of expired air for hydrogen or isotopically tagged CO after administration of lactulose (H_2), labeled bile acids (^{14}C-cholylglycine), or labeled xylose (CO_2). The procedure is dependent on the availability of a breath analyzer. There is a problem with the differentiation of small intestinal from colonic bacteria which will happily metabolize the test compounds. There are false-negatives as well as false-positives. Nonetheless, the ease of performance, particularly for serial studies, and the patient acceptability probably make this the test of choice both for screening and follow-up, as long as the test's limitations are observed and respected (King & Toskes, 1979; Davidson, et al., 1984).

The ideal critical path for the diagnosis would include suspicion of bacterial overgrowth, evaluation for predisposing anatomical or physiological abnormality, screening breath test, quantitative culture if there is a positive breath test, treatment, and post-treatment follow-up with breath tests. When a predisposing cause is clear and a screening breath test is positive, appropriate management may well be to skip the culture and proceed with antibiotics.

Treatment

Treatment should include nutritional support to restore the nutritional deficits. Selection of the form and the route of the supplement depend on the definitive therapy selected. If there is an anatomical defect that can be eliminated surgically or a physiological defect that can be corrected with medical therapy, then this is curative treatment and the treatment of choice. More often than not, these options are not open. The alternative is to attempt to eliminate or control the overgrowth with antimicrobial therapy. Interestingly, because the flora is usually very complex, routine sensitivity studies of cultured organisms have not proven worthwhile. A trial of tetracycline, 250 mg four times daily for two weeks, is customary. Response in terms of reduction in diarrhea and improved absorption should be evident within one week and often within one day. Failure to respond may imply the wrong diagnosis, but a drug-resistant flora is a more likely explanation. Second line drugs, including chloramphenicol, lincomycin, metronidazole, and clindamycin, have all been used with success. Use of antibiotics should be limited to a definite course of therapy and as few of these as it takes to control symptoms in order to limit the emergence of antibiotic-resistant flora. Failure of this approach should prompt referral to a center equipped to perform quantitative anaerobic culture with isolation and antibiotic sensitivity studies (King & Toskes, 1979).

Interim nutritional support, mentioned above, must be tailored to the degree of the patient's malnutrition as well as the effectiveness of therapy in the correction of the malabsorption. Elimination of lactose from the diet and the use of medium chain triglycerides will be of importance in the presurgical patient and in the patient slow to respond to medical therapy (King & Toskes, 1979).

Syndromes of Intestinal Obstruction

Small intestinal obstruction can be the end result of many diverse intestinal problems (Table 3–2). None of these is really a phenomenon of aging, but all represent problems that tend to accumulate in the

TABLE 3–2. Syndromes of Small Intestinal Obstruction

Inflammatory stricture	Mechanical obstruction
Crohn's disease	Hernia
Acute and chronic small bowel ulcer	Gallstone ileus
Postirradiation	Tumor
Acute vascular occlusion	Intussusception
Cicatrix	Diabetic visceral neuropathy
Crohn's disease	Pseudo-obstruction
Healed(ing) ulcer	
Healed(ing) vascular occlusion	

elderly population. The presentation and management of intestinal obstruction in the elderly demand little difference from that in a younger patient of similar general health and with equivalent complicating problems. The numbers of frail patients with limited tolerance and reserve are higher among the elderly, and thus as a group they are harder to manage. The patterns of ocurrence of the various etiologies do change in the elderly group, and there is some diagnostic advantage in knowing these differences.

Crohn's Disease

With improvement in therapy, a significant number of patients with Crohn's disease survive to old age. In addition, ten percent or more of Crohn's patients have the onset of their disease after age 60 (Goligher, 1968). Acute and chronic obstruction can be complications that require Crohn's disease to be included in the differential diagnosis of intestinal obstruction in the elderly.

Ulceration

Small intestinal ulcers are uncommon, and most are found in the elderly. Their true frequency is unknown because they are located in a region blind to most of our diagnostic maneuvers, and only a complication brings attention to the ulcer. Most of the ulcers occur in the ileum. Although fewer ulcers occur in the jejunum, in this location they seem more likely to perforate. Bleeding and intestinal obstruction are the usual attention-getting clinical events. The underlying cause of the complication is often not recognized until operation (Boydstun, et al., 1981). The etiologies of the ulcerations are many, including Crohn's disease, vascular insufficiency, tumor, gluten-sensitive enteropathy, drug-induced lesions, and a large percentage that remains idiopathic.

Drug-induced ulcers currently seem related to slow release forms of indomethacin, but it is likely that, as other slow release forms of medications become available, this list will grow. The large number of idiopathic lesions must include a number of differing mechanisms. In the absence of a treatable cause, definitive therapy is surgical. Published mortality rates are 8.5 per cent, which serve to underline the seriousness of these ulcers (Boydstun, et al., 1981).

Radiation Enteritis

Gluten-sensitive enteropathy, tumors, diabetic neuropathy, and vascular insufficiency are discussed elsewhere in this chapter. Chronic changes following pelvic irradiation, often long in the past, can lead to partial or complete obstruction. Here, because of the adhesions and the matting together of loops of bowel, surgical intervention is often formidable and to be avoided if possible. Nutritional support and the treatment of bacterial overgrowth to reduce diarrhea will often permit one to avoid or delay surgery (Novak, et al., 1979).

Intestinal Pseudo-obstruction

Pseudo-obstruction syndrome is the final common path for many diverse problems. The patient presents with all the signs and symptoms of small intestinal obstruction, but careful evaluation reveals no anatomical evidence of an obstructing lesion. Obstruction may involve any hollow viscus, including the bladder. The site of the obstruction may be sharply localized or general. The primary disease, characterized by chronic and recurrent attacks, may afflict any age group. The elderly seem particularly susceptible to the secondary form, which is often acute and frequently has a diagnosis associated with a primary problem. Table 3–3 lists the secondary causes of pseudo-obstruction as outlined by Faulk, Anuras, and Christensen (1978). To this list should be added

TABLE 3–3. Chronic Intestinal Pseudo-obstruction: Secondary Causes

Diseases involving the intestinal smooth muscle	Neurological diseases
Collagen-vascular diseases	Parkinson's disease
Scleroderma	Hirschsprung's disease
Dermatomyositis/polymyositis	Chagas' disease
Systemic lupus erythematosus	Familial autonomic dysfunction
Amyloidosis	**Pharmacological causes**
Primary muscle diseases	Phenothiazines
Myotonic dystrophy	Tricyclic antidepressants
Progressive muscular dystrophy	Antiparkinsonian medications
Ceroidosis	Ganglionic blockers
Nontropical sprue	Clonidine
Endocrine disorders	*Anamita* (mushroom) poisoning
Myxedema	Miscellaneous
Diabetes	Jejunoileal bypass
Hypoparathyroidism	Diverticulosis (jejunal)
Pheochromocytoma	Psychosis
	Cathartic colon

the transient obstruction that can accompany chronic congestive heart failure, chronic renal failure, and other diseases associated with hypokalemia, hypochloridemia, and hypomagnesemia. Funtional obstruction is also associated with remote inflammation, either major sepsis or the inflammation that occurs with pancreatitis or cholecystitis.

Clinical Management

Management of the problem always starts with the management of the acute obstruction. Particular attention has to be paid to fluid and electrolyte balance in the elderly in whom the tolerance for overload is apt to be compromised by other intercurrent or preexisting problems. When acute problems are stabilized, full attention should be paid to the underlying cause.

Crohn's Disease (Inflammatory Bowel Disease, Regional Ileitis)

Two features combine to make Crohn's disease a problem in the elderly. First, Crohn's has been the focus of much study that has resulted in significant progress in the management of the disease. Management is still far from optimal, with a limited formulary at hand and a frequent need to resort to surgical intervention; but on the whole, patients are living longer, avoiding the many complications, and successfully entering the geriatric age group. A second feature is the appreciation that ten per cent or more of patients with Crohn's disease have their first attack after age 60. Many studies have emphasized epidemiological evidence for a small secondary peak in the incidence of Crohn's disease in the 60 to 70 year age group (Goligher, et al., 1968; Harper, et al., 1986).

As has been mentioned for several other diseases, there is little information to suggest that the course of the disease differs in the elderly from that in younger age groups if one makes allowances for the patient's general condition and other unassociated diseases. When these are added in, the elderly do in fact face an increased morbidity and mortality from Crohn's disease.

The clinical diagnosis is based on the same features of history, physical, laboratory, and x-ray examinations for young and old alike. The hallmarks of the presentation include fever and abdominal pain. Diarrhea with Crohn's disease suggests but is not pathognomonic of ileocolitis. Separation from ischemic disease and from diverticulitis are major problems in the differential diagnosis.

Medical management requires added caution in the elderly. Sulfasalazine seems well tolerated, but corticosteroids, while effective, are apt to exacerbate problems with osteoporosis, diabetes, and other intercurrent problems. The key to successful use of steroids seems to rest with the use of adequate doses for the shortest possible time necessary to control the disease process. The steroid sparing effect of the addition of an immunosuppressant such as azothioprine or 6-mercaptopurine would be attractive in this setting; however, many elderly patients prove to have an unusually sensitive response to immunosuppressives which complicates their use.

The indications for surgery remain the same regardless of age. Surgery is not curative but rather is one more step in the progression of the disease. Unfortunately, this has led many clinicians to delay surgical intervention, adding to the morbidity and the patient's suffering. The margin for the tolerance of the disease process in the elderly may be narrowed, and thus the timing of surgical intervention is critical.

Neoplasms

With advancing age, the small intestine shares with the rest of the gastrointestinal tract the increasing incidence of the development of tumors. The small intestine is a minor participant, with the smallest numbers of tumors, benign or malignant, in the digestive tract. The spectrum of benign tumors—lipoma, leiomyoma, hemangioma, and adenoma—is unchanged by age. Most of these tumors are silent clinically. Occasionally one will bleed or form the leading point of an intussusception.

Malignant tumors include carcinomas, carcinoid, leiomyosarcoma, and lymphoma, and these more often become symptomatic. In spite of the production of symptoms, the diagnosis is never easy. The small intestine is difficult to visualize with any testing modality. The most common malignant tumor is a metastatic lesion. The behavior and treatment of these malignant lesions are the same in the elderly as in younger patients. The most common primary tumor is a carcinoid. A functioning carcinoid is easily diagnosed by measuring 5HIAA levels. Sadly, the diagnosis of a functioning carcinoid implies that it has already metastasized to the liver. Nonfunctioning carcinoids and other malignant tumors of the small intestine usually present with intestinal obstruction or bleeding. Unfortunately, this also is usually too late in the natural history of the tumor to offer much hope for surgical cure, and the prognosis is therefore poor (Barclay & Schapira, 1983).

Vascular Disease

Ischemic disease as a result of age-related alterations in and to the arterial supply and the venous drainage of the small and large intestine are infrequent, but far from rare, problems of the elderly. When ischemic problems do occur, they tend to present as catastrophes. Early, aggressive management can do much to lower morbidity and mortality, but a high level of suspicion and good diagnostic judgment are needed to achieve early intervention. There are many ways to try to classify the various forms of ischemic disease that affect the intestine. Most of these classifications stumble over the discrepancy between the anatomical site of the primary lesion, embolus or thrombus, and the resultant site of damage to the intestine.

Anatomy

Three vessels feed the intestinal tract. These are the celiac plexus (Fig. 3–2) with its branches (left gastric, splenic, and hepatic arteries). The anterior and posterior pancreatoduodenal arteries carry hepatic arterial blood through a series of arcades to feed the duodenum, and these arcades anastomose with arcades of the superior mesenteric artery drainage. The second major branch of the aorta that supplies the intestine is the superior mesenteric artery (Fig. 3–3), which branches to form the inferior pancreatoduodenal, the right colic, the middle colic, the ileocolic, and the intestinal arteries, twelve to sixteen in number. These arteries supply the intestine from the lower part of the duodenum to the mid-transverse colon. As these arteries pass toward the intestine, they branch and the branches inosculate to form a series of arcades. Where the course of the artery is short, only a single arcade is formed. Where the course takes a longer journey through the mesentery two, three, four, or even five levels of such arcades can be formed. The third major artery is the inferior mesenteric artery (Fig. 3–4) with its branches (left colic, sigmoid, and superior hemorrhoidal arteries). These all feed the colon from the mid-transverse colon through the rectum. These arteries also form arcades, and those of the left colic inosculate freely with the arcades of the superior mesenteric artery (Ruzicka & Rossi, 1970; Schaeffer, 1942).

Pathophysiology

Anastomotic Channels

In the event of an occlusion—complete or incomplete, chronic or acute—the immediate response is to open this extensive system of anastomotic channels and to bypass the area of obstructed arterial flow. Where the occlusion is gradual in onset, these anastomotic channels can enlarge to replace even major occluded vessels. Often this includes the enlargement of the marginal artery of Drummond and/or the arc of Ridon which can form the wandering mesenteric artery. There are

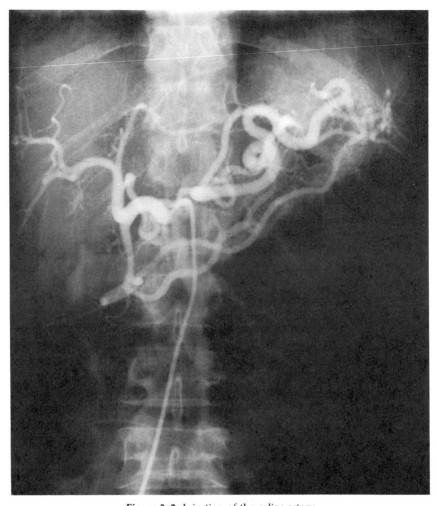

Figure 3–2. Injection of the celiac artery.

many reports in the literature of asymptomatic patients with total occlusion of all three arteries.

Perfusion

Even when the occlusion is acute, it is still possible for the anastomotic connections to provide adequate perfusion to maintain viable intestine. The wall of the intestine harbors a network of interconnecting capillary beds, many of which are not perfused in the resting state. The rule of thumb has been that in the resting intestine at any given time only 20 per cent of the capillary bed requires perfusion; thus, if anastomotic channels can maintain only 20 per cent of the usual

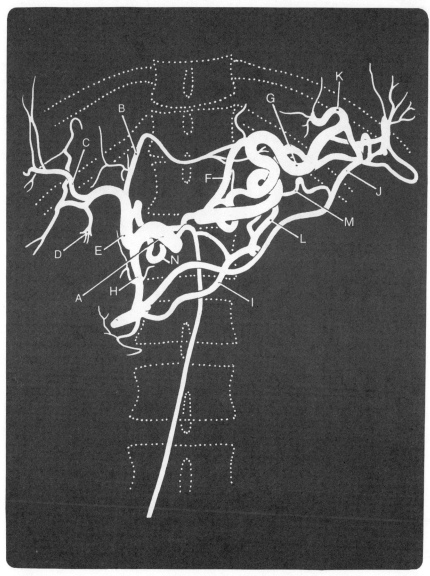

Figure 3–2 *Continued*

A Celiac artery
B Left hepatic artery
C Right hepatic artery
D Cystic artery
E Common hepatic artery
F Left gastric artery
G Splenic artery

H Gastroduodenal artery
I Gastroepiploic artery right
J Gastroepiploic artery left
K Short gastric artery
L Dorsal pancreatic artery
M Pancreatic magna
N Pancreatoduodenal artery branch

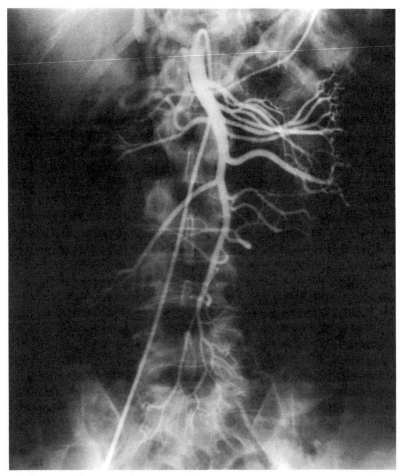

Figure 3–3. Injection of the superior mesenteric artery.

blood flow, the bowel can remain viable (Brandt, 1984). However, function may be severely compromised.

Much of the occlusive disease, both chronic and acute, that involves intestinal vasculature is located close to the origin of the arteries from the aorta. Major mesenteric arteries do not resemble the end arteries of the brain or the myocardium where occlusion results in a predictable pattern of damage. Here the system is better likened to the plumbing in an aging apartment building. Because of interconnections in the pipes, a sudden change in flow in one part of the system may well result in an unanticipated change in the flow in remote apartments that share the same water system. Pity the plumber who must identify and

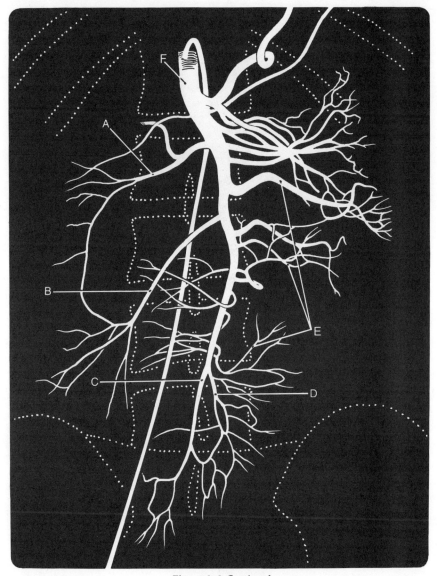

Figure 3–3 *Continued*

A Middle colic artery
B Right colic artery
C Ileocolic artery

D Ileal artery
E Jejunal artery
F Superior mesenteric artery

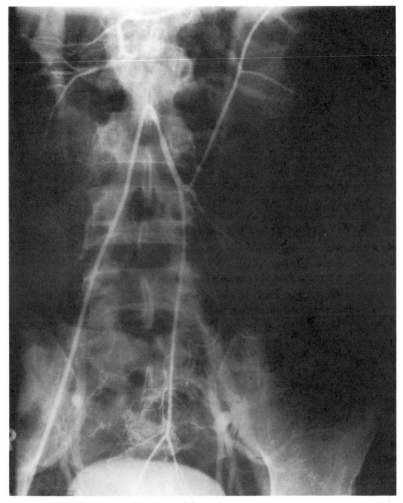

Figure 3–4. Injection of the inferior mesenteric artery.

repair the site of significant obstruction wherever it is before he can restore the flow in a given apartment.

Secondary Vasospasm

An additional factor in the diagnosis and management of intestinal vascular disease is the role that vasospasm plays in the development and progression of the ischemic lesion. An acute occlusion results in rapid opening of anastomotic channels to restore perfusion. As this process approaches equilibrium, and if the perfusion pressure distal to the occlusion remains low, the involved vascular bed responds with vasoconstriction (Boley, et al., 1969; Brant & Boley, 1981). Generally in

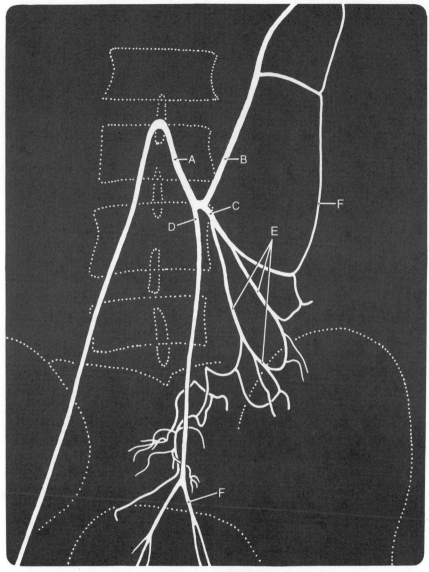

Figure 3–4 *Continued*

A Inferior mesenteric artery
B Left colic artery—ascending branch
C Left colic artery

D Superior hemorrhoidal artery
E Sigmoid arteries
F Marginal artery of Drummond

cases of nonocclusive ischemia, there is a systemic circulatory problem, such as congestive heart failure, that results in a fall in perfusion. Again vasoconstriction is a response to enhance the pressure of what perfusion does occur. When this vasoconstriction persists for more than several hours, as little as two hours in some patients but more often four, then relief of the obstruction or restoration of perfusion does not relieve the vasoconstriction. This is a working explanation for the progression of ischemic lesions in the face of surgical or medical restoration of perfusion and, as it turns out, is much of the working basis of the programs for aggressive intervention in management of these problems (Brandt, 1984).

Acute Hypoperfusion

Acute ischemic bowel infarction is a major life-threatening emergency. In simplest terms, it represents underperfusion of a segment of the intestine past the limit of viability of the bowel wall. The natural evolution of the lesion is the development of gangrene of the intestinal wall, perforation, peritonitis, and death. Early recognition would permit restoration of perfusion before the loss of viability of the bowel wall. Failing this, the dead bowel must be resected and circulation restored to the remaining bowel.

Clinical Presentation

Clinically the presentation begins with pain. At the outset this pain is colicky with the traditional small intestinal reference point, the umbilicus. As the infarction progresses, the pain becomes less colicky and more generalized. Distention and its fellow traveler, vomiting, are also early features. These both represent some degree of functional obstruction secondary to spasm of intestinal musculature. Hematemesis and hematochezia occur. Early in the infarction, these complaints of pain and distention are out of proportion to the physical findings on examination of the abdomen. The signs of peritoneal irritation with rebound tenderness or rigidity await the maturation of the infarction. While mild fever can occur early in the course, high temperatures and leucocytosis are also late findings. Prior to the occurrence of irreversibly dead bowel, most of the changes in laboratory values are nonspecific and do not particularly suggest infarction of the bowel.

Radiological Findings

Radiological studies provide much more diagnostic insight. Flat and upright films of the abdomen are likely starting points for investigation. Frequently, these have little to add; however, there are occasional diagnostic findings. The absence of a gas pattern early in the course of an infarction is one such finding. This is a result of intense spasm of small intestine musculature (Marston, 1977). Later in the course, as distention becomes a feature, gas appears on the plain film. If the gas pattern shows a cutoff at the junction of the superior and inferior mesenteric arteries distribution (for practical purposes at the splenic flexure), this can be of great diagnostic aid (Tomchick, 1970). Thickening of the bowel wall, gas in the bowel wall, and gas present in the portal venous system are also helpful clues.

The decision concerning the use of barium contrast studies or angiography as diagnostic tools is in dispute. One body of opinion holds that angiography is employed after the diagnosis is made, both to confirm the diagnosis and to prospect for a repairable lesion (Spiro, 1983). The other side of the controversy includes the aggressive management school which would utilize angiography much earlier, in effect screening for the diagnosis in patients presenting with abdominal pain for which ischemia is in the differential diagnosis (Brandt, 1984). This is more than a semantic splitting of hairs. The aggressive interventionists maintain that clinical signs which permit a firm diagnosis are equated with dead bowel in the peritoneal cavity, and if one wishes to avoid infarction or at best to minimize it, it takes early demonstration of the obstruction or the poor perfusion to permit optimal management. They maintain that angiograms are safe and of low morbidity even in the very ill patient and that in some circumstances the catheter can be used in therapy (Brandt, 1984). The more conservative school is unwilling to accept the number of screening angiograms necessary to identify treatable lesions. This represents a cost in morbidity, in delayed diagnosis of other problems, in resources, and in dollars which perhaps is not yet justified.

Clearly there are elements of truth in both arguments, which means that there is not yet a standard protocol to follow and each patient's care must be individualized. When the clinical history and the background suggest embolus as a possibility (atrial fibrillation, myocardial infarction, rheumatic valvular heart disease, or prosthetic valves are all predisposers), then angiography with an eye toward embolectomy is the first choice. When all predisposing conditions seem lacking, the use of barium contrast studies as well as other studies to search for an as yet undefined abdominal catastrophe is in order. The diagnostic pathway in a patient whose history suggests nonobstructive hypoperfusion is not so clear. The emerging success of the direct infusion of vasodilators into the superior mesenteric artery rather tips the scale toward angiography.

The diagnostic features for ischemic bowel on barium enema include the combination of hyperirritability usually manifest as spasm and thumbprinting, which represents the development of focal mucosal edema and hemorrhage.

Treatment

Management is by restoration of perfusion and resection of dead bowel where necessary. Even where there is a clear need for surgical intervention to remove an embolus or an obstructing lesion, the use of medical support to control vasospasm is in order (Brandt & Boley, 1981). It seems likely that innovative tools in the management of these problems will emerge as the percutaneous applications of the laser, the rongeur, and the balloon dilator are exploited. These will in turn reinforce the diagnostic importance of the angiogram.

Chronic Hypoperfusion

Chronic ischemia is responsible for two well-recognized clinical syndromes: intestinal angina and malabsorption. Both syndromes find their pathophysiological roots in the necessary vascular response to the ingestion of a meal. Transit, digestion, and absorption are the work of the intestinal tract and obligate significant increases in vascular perfusion in the performance of this work. While progressive atherosclerosis is the most common cause, one also needs to remember that chronic hypoperfusion has been associated with aneurysm involving the aorta or the larger abdominal vessels and arteriovenous fistulas. The occurrence of malabsorption as a complication of chronic ischemia is often mentioned in discussions of malabsorption but receives little if any discussion in presentations on mesenteric vascular disease. It is not a common clinical manifestation of ischemia (Shaw & Maynard, 1959).

Intestinal angina clinically presents as postprandial crampy abdominal discomfort that comes on in the first half hour after a meal and persists for several hours. The size of the meal required to bring on the pain varies from patient to patient, and the individual patient quickly develops a sensitivity to this feature. The other characteristic finding is weight loss, usually attributed to a reluctance to eat but which may in part be due to malabsorption. This pattern of abdominal pain and wasting in an elderly patient leads to much concern over the presence of a malignancy and often delays the diagnosis of chronic ischemia. Sutton's law suggests that this delay is appropriate and necessary since intraabdominal malignancy is far more common in the elderly than is intestinal angina.

The diagnosis is confirmed by angiographic evidence of impaired flow (Brant & Boley, 1981). Management depends on the patient's condition. Medically one can use multiple small feedings in an attempt to restore nutrition. If this fails, the alternatives are parenteral alimentation, with some undesirable risks and costs, or attempts at vascular reconstructive surgery. Surgery too has some risks, but if the angiograms suggest that reconstruction is feasible, this is an elegant solution.

One hopes that a percutaneous procedure—laser, rongeur, or balloon dilatation—may find a role in treatment of this lesion.

Focal Vascular Lesions in the Small Intestine (Small Vessel Disease)

A host of problems with widely different etiologies hides under the general category of focal or small vessel disease. The outline in Table 3–4 lists most of the common associated etiologies. There is an equally long list of uncommon purpuras and inheritable conditions that seem to predispose to focal vascular disease. Most of these are not particular problems of the elderly. Atherosclerosis, adhesions with the opportunity for strangulation, and radiation injury are examples of problems that do accumulate in an aging population. Improved management of collagen-vascular diseases accounts for an increased number of afflicted elderly. The first key to diagnosis rests with awareness of the range of diagnoses predisposing to focal ischemia.

Clinical Presentation

The small intestine has a limited spectrum of responses. These include infarction of the bowel wall with or without gangrene and perforation, deep ulceration (extending through the submucosa), mucosal ulceration, bleeding, ileus, and scarring with partial or complete stricture as the lesion resolves. The problem may be acute in onset with rapid evolution, in which case the diagnostic dilemma is that of an acute abdomen. A strangulation due to torsion about an adhesion is the best example of an acute lesion. It may also be slow in both onset and evolution, such as what occurs in arteriosclerotic disease. If changes are slow enough, the disease may only become apparent in the form

TABLE 3–4. Focal and Small Vessel Intestinal Ischemia

Strangulated hernia
Adhesions with strangulation of a loop of bowel
Trauma to the mesentery
Atherosclerosis
Malignant hypertension
Radiation injury
Inflammatory bowel disease
Mesenteric arteritis after repair of a coarctation of the aorta
Degos' disease
Ergot ingestion
Collagen-vascular diseases (immune-complex diseases)
   Systemic lupus erythematosus
   Rheumatoid arthritis
   Scleroderma
   Periarteritis nodosa
   Dermatomyositis
   Schönlein-Henoch purpura

of a complication such as bacterial overgrowth behind a partial stricture. Radiation damage may have both an acute and a chronic component.

Two other features must also be considered as determinants of the clinical presentation. These are the positioning of the focal lesion and the linear extent of the lesion or lesions, since they can be multiple. Lesions high in the jejunum are more likely to be associated with vomiting and, if the problem is chronic, to more profoundly impair general nutrition than are distal lesions. The greater the aggregate length of the intestine that is involved, the more likely that it will produce symptoms.

Diagnosis and Management

Diagnosis of most of these problems rests with ruling in or ruling out the presence of an acute abdomen and relating it to an associated or predisposing illness or, in the case of chronic lesions, the recognition of a specific intestinal lesion against the background of a chronic systemic disease. Management includes specific therapy for the underlying problem if there is one as well as therapy directed toward the intestinal lesion. Dead bowel must be resected. Strictures likewise must be approached surgically if the patient's condition permits. Most of the other focal problems in the small intestine are difficult and often impossible to localize by noninvasive methods. It is tempting to suggest that healing should be accelerated by placing the bowel at rest and thus eliminating the food-related demand for increased vascular perfusion. Unfortunately, while it is a common-sense approach, there are little data to justify parenteral alimentation especially given its risks and costs. One is faced with surgical treatment of abdominal emergencies or medical therapy of underlying systemic ills in the hope that the intestinal lesion improves before a complicating emergency intervenes.

Venous Thrombosis

Acute thrombosis in the mesenteric veins is an infrequent but well-recognized cause of intestinal infarction. Associated conditions are listed on Table 3–5 as prepared by Grendell and Ockner (1982). Many are idiopathic. Well-recognized causes include contiguous spread of local intraabdominal inflammation. Appendicitis, pyelonephritis, and inflamed colonic diverticulum are leading offenders, although any intraabdominal inflammation can serve as a cause. Mesenteric venous thrombosis is a recognized complication of hypercoagulation states of whatever cause, and as one would expect, venous congestion (such as is associated with cirrhosis) also predisposes. Trauma (including surgical trauma) can also result in venous thrombosis. There is little mention of drug-related thrombosis now, although in years gone by

TABLE 3–5. Conditions Associated with Mesenteric Venous Thrombosis

Portal hypertension
   Cirrhosis
   Congestive splenomegaly
Inflammation
   Peritonitis (e.g., appendicitis, perforated viscus)
   Inflammatory bowel disease
   Pelvic or intraabdominal abscess
   Diverticular disease
Postoperative state and trauma
   Splenectomy and other postoperative states
   Blunt abdominal trauma*
"Hypercoagulable" states
   Neoplasms (especially intraabdominal—e.g., colonic or pancreatic)
   Oral contraceptive use
   Pregnancy*
   Migratory thrombophlebitis
   Antithrombin III deficiency
   Peripheral deep vein thrombosis
   Polycythemia vera
   Thrombocytosis
Other conditions
   Renal disease (including kidney transplantation*)
   Cardiac disease

*Rare, isolated reports
Reprinted with permission from Grendell, J. H., and Ockner, R. K.: Mesenteric venous thrombosis. Gastroenterology 82:358–392, 1982. Copyright 1982 by the American Gastroenterological Association.

enteric-coated potassium was implicated as a cause of venous thrombosis. The slow release and enteric-coated forms of some nonsteroidal anti-inflammatory agents are associated with the development of small intestinal ulcers, but it is not clear whether the drug acts directly on the mucosa or through a vascular mechanism.

Clinically, these lesions often do not present as acute abdominal emergencies and are rather more indolent in onset. As in all infarctions, abdominal pain is the common complaint. The duration of pain may be days, weeks, or months. Since the vascular obstruction is venous in location, congestion is the immediate result. The involved bowel wall becomes edematous, and there is transudation, usually into the lumen, with consequent distention. A concomitant decrease in motility adds to the distention. Clinical dehydration may be evident. Congestion of the bowel wall may proceed to the point of necrosis with bleeding into the lumen and/or the development of peritoneal signs. Preoperative diagnosis is a coup. Most often the diagnosis does not become apparent until the patient is operated on for a presumed acute abdomen.

Plain x-rays can show ileus with thickening of the bowel wall and thumbprinting. If one is perceptive enough to order an angiogram, it will show a delayed or absent venous phase and often difficulty in filling the superior mesenteric artery (Grendell & Ockner, 1982).

Management at operation includes resection of any infarcted bowel as well as, where feasible, tending to the primary cause. Postoperative management includes the use of anticoagulants to prevent recurrent thrombosis.

REFERENCES

Anuras, S., et al.: Intestinal pseudoobstruction. Gastroenterology 74:1318–1324, 1978.
Anuras, S., and Sutherland, J.: Jejunal manometry in healthy elderly subjects. Gastroenterology 86:1016, 1984.
Baer, A.N., et al.: Intestinal ulceration and malabsorption syndromes. Gastroenterology 79:754–765, 1980.
Barclay, T.H.C., and Schapira, D.V.: Malignant tumors of the small intestine. Cancer 51:878–881, 1983.
Batt, R.M., et al.: Biochemical changes in the jejunal mucosa of dogs with a naturally occurring enteropathy associated with bacterial overgrowth. Gut 25:816–823, 1984.
Boley, S.J., et al.: Circulatory responses to acute reduction of superior mesenteric arterial flow. Physiologist 12:180, 1969.
Boydstun, J.S., Jr., et al.: Clinicopathologic study of nonspecific ulcers of the small intestine. Dig Dis Sci 26:911–916, 1981.
Brandt, L.J.: Gastrointestinal Disorders of the Elderly. New York, Raven Press, 1984.
Brandt, L.J., and Boley, S.J.: Ischemic intestinal syndromes. Adv Surg 15:1–45, 1981.
Davidson, G.P., et al.: Bacterial contamination of the small intestine as an important cause of chronic diarrhea and abdominal pain: Diagnosis by breath hydrogen test. Pediatrics 74:229–235, 1984.
Faulk, D.L., et al.: Chronic intestinal pseudoobstruction. Gastroenterology 74:922–931, 1978.
Fedorak, R.N., et al.: Treatment of diabetic diarrhea with clonidine. Ann Intern Med 102:197–199, 1985.
Feibusch, J., and Holt, P.R.: Impaired absorptive capacity for carbohydrates in the elderly. Am J Clin Nutr 32:942, 1979.
Grendell, J.H., and Ockner, P.K.: Mesenteric venous thrombosis. Gastroenterology 82:358–392, 1982.
Goligher, J.D., et al.: Ulcerative Colitis. London, Balliere, Tindall and Cassell, 1968.
Goyal, R.K., and Spiro, H.M.: Gastrointestinal manifestations of diabetes mellitus. Med Clin North Am 59:1031–1044, 1971.
Harper, P.C., et al.: Crohn's disease in the elderly: A statistical comparison with younger patients matched for sex and duration of disease. Arch Intern Med 146:753–755, 1986.
Holmes, G.K.T., et al.: Coeliac disease, gluten free diet and malignancy. Gut 17:612–619, 1976.
Holt, P.R.: The small intestine. Clin Gastroenterol 14:689–723, 1985.
King, C.E., and Toskes, P.P.: Small intestine bacterial overgrowth. Gastroenterology 76:1035–1055, 1979.
Marston, A.: Intestinal Ischemia. Chicago, Yearbook Medical Publishers, 1977.
McEvoy, A., et al.: Bacterial contamination of the small intestine is an important cause of occult malabsorption in the elderly. Br Med J 287:789–793, 1983.
Novak, J., et al.: Effects of radiation on the human gastrointestinal tract. J Clin Gastroenterol 1:9–39, 1979.
Roberts, S.H., et al: Bacterial overgrowth syndrome without "blind loop": A cause for malnutrition in the elderly. Lancet 2:1193–1195, 1977.
Ruzicka, F.F., and Rossi, P.: Normal vascular anatomy of the abdominal viscera. Radiol Clin North Am 8:3–29, 1970.
Schaeffer, J.P.: Morris' Human Anatomy. 11th ed. Toronto, The Blakiston Company, 1942.

Schneider, E.L., et al.: Recommended dietary allowances and the health of the elderly. N Engl J Med 314:157–160, 1986.

Shaw, R.S., and Maynard, E.P.: Acute and chronic thrombosis of the mesenteric arteries associated with malabsorption: A report of two cases successfully treated by thromboendarectomy. N Engl Med 258:874–878, 1959.

Simon, G.L., and Gorbach, S.L.: Intestinal flora in health and disease. Gastroenterology 1:174–193, 1984.

Spiro, H.M.: Clinical Gastroenterology. New York, Macmillan Publishing Co., 1983.

Swinson, C.M., and Levi, A.J.: Is coeliac disease underdiagnosed? Br Med J 281:1258–1260, 1980.

Tomchik, F.S., et al.: The roentgenographic spectrum of bowel infarction. Radiology 96:249–260, 1970.

VanTrappen, G., et al.: The interdigestive motor complex of normal subjects and patients with bacterial overgrowth of the small intestine. J Clin Invest 59:1158–1166, 1977.

Webster, S.G.P., and Leeming, J.T.: The appearance of the small bowel mucosa in old age. Age Aging 4:168–174, 1975.

Webster, S.G.P., and Leeming, J.T.: Assessment of small bowel function in the elderly using a modified xylose tolerance test. Gut 16:109–113, 1975.

Whalen, G.E., et al.: Diabetic diarrhea. A clinical and pathophysiological study. Gastroenterology 56:1021–1032, 1969.

Chapter 4
NORMAL COLON FUNCTION AND AGING

William A. Sodeman, Jr.

The large intestine is host to a number of disease processes in the elderly which have long been considered to be problems related to the aging of the intestinal musculature and of its integration. Most of these disease processes now appear to involve environmental influences that take time and/or a long exposure for their development rather than a result of changes secondary to the aging of intestinal muscle alone. It should be of no surprise if, in fact, it is the interaction between both the aging process and the environment which underlies many of these problems. Diverticular disease, muscular thickening of the sigmoid, angiodysplasia in the colon, and carcinoma of the colon are perhaps the best examples. Heedless of the mechanism, the end result is a focus of geriatric problems involving the colon.

NORMAL PHYSIOLOGY

The large intestine is primarily involved in salt and water homeostasis. It has little role in the absorption of nutrients under normal circumstances, and few substances require excretion across the colonic mucosa. Recovery of salt and water from the nonabsorbable residue in the intestine followed by elimination of this residue is a very early

79

phylogenetic development. Evolution of the colonic mechanisms necessary to accomplish this are closely related to the composition of the diet. Recent changes (recent on an evolutionary time scale) in foodstuffs and their processing have resulted in disturbed colon and rectal function to, or perhaps, beyond the physiological limits. In addition, social and hygienic necessity has forced a voluntary, reservoir function upon the colon—a function that evolutionary change may not have provided for.

The functional design of the esophagus facilitates rapid transit of liquids and solids to the stomach. The stomach acts as a reservoir adjusting the tonicity of ingested food and furthering the digestive process with acid and enzymes. The diluted chyme is released into the small intestine in small volumes at a feedback controlled rate. Passage down the small intestine with further digestion and absorption of nutrients is rapid, with the residue of one's lunch arriving at the ileocecal valve at the time one's supper is ingested. Passage through the esophagus takes seconds, through the stomach minutes, and through the small intestine hours. Passage through the colon takes days. Some slowing of colonic transit is necessary to permit dehydration of the fecal mass and absorption of electrolytes. The motility mechanisms and their pattern of action differ in the colon from patterns observed elsewhere in the digestive tract.

Motility and Transit

The wall of the colon has four layers: mucosa, submucosa, muscularis propria,and serosa. The mucosal surface is not comprised of villus-like folds as is the small intestine; rather it is flat with polygonal units delineated by shallow clefts (Fig. 4–1). Goblet cells open onto the surface, and a crypt of Lieberkühn opens in the center of each polygonal unit. The muscularis propria consists of an inner layer of circular muscle and an outer layer of longitudinal muscle. The longitudinally arranged muscle covers the entire surface of the colon, but it is gathered at three points into thickened bands—the teniae—which run the length of the colon. The longitudinal muscle bridging the space between the teniae is thinned and nonfunctional. The circular muscle is arranged in overlapping, semicircular fasciculi that are firmly connected to the teniae. The teniae serve in part as a kind of skeleton from which the fasciculi of circular muscle are hung. Contraction of the teniae affords some structural integrity during the contraction of the circular muscles. If the system is functioning optimally, contraction of the teniae will be limited to a degree of tension necessary to stabilize a colonic segment during a motility event. This degree of contraction will be greater when the colon is empty (compressing like an accordion) than when it is filled with intestinal content. In addition, shortening the colon by teniae

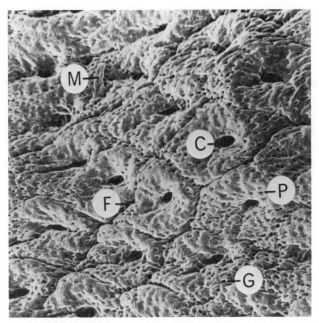

Figure 4–1. A view of the normal rectal mucosa obtained with a scanning electron microscope. Each crypt (C) opens on the surface in the center of a polygonal unit defined by a furrow (F). Empty (G) and filled (P) goblet cells are visible. X 240. (Used with the permission of Kavin H, Hamilton DG, et al.: Scanning electron microscopy. Gastroenterology 59:427, 1970.)

contraction throws the mucosa into broad transverse folds that may partially occlude the lumen.

Contraction of fasciculi of circular muscle increases tension in the wall and pressure on the intestinal content. This increased pressure is usually focal and creates a pressure differential that results in net movement of intestinal contents up and/or down the lumen of the colon—the direction is governed by that of the intralumenal pressure gradient. Observations suggest that wall tensions necessary to achieve a gradient are smaller as the colonic lumen fills with intestinal content. As the volume of lumenal content falls, there is the possibility of development of a contraction sufficient to produce closed chambers in the colon with the potential development of high pressures and wall tensions in the closed chamber.

The movement of intestinal contents has proven technically difficult to study. The net movements of colonic content are slow with transit measured in days, but the local propulsive events are often of short duration with long quiescent intervals. It requires long-study intervals to identify critical motility events. The integration of the motility mechanisms to produce controlled transit is responsive to a variety of neural and humoral influences. An intact intrinsic innervation is essential for an orderly process. A number of motility events have been observed including haustral shuttling, haustral propulsion and retropulsion, systolic and serial multihaustral propulsion, peristaltic ripples, peristalsis, and mass movement (Ritchie, 1971). The apparent pattern of the motility event is probably a function of the length of the colonic segment integrated into the process.

An overlooked feature of the mechanisms of motility is the importance of gravity and/or physical activity. It is a time-hallowed observation that hospitalization of a patient is associated with slowing of the frequency of bowel movements. It is not clear whether rest or the supine posture is responsible, but both are suspect. Any significant change in lifestyle toward inactivity seems to be accompanied by sluggish bowel action. It is also not clear whether the effect involves colonic transit or the process of defecation. While the problem is well recognized, it remains so poorly understood from the standpoint of pathophysiology that it is usually only mentioned in passing. It is probably a significant cause of perturbed colonic function in the elderly.

Disturbance of the normal motility process underlies many of the colonic diseases associated with aging. The aging process itself produces some morphological and histological changes in the colonic musculature. There is from birth a gradual thickening of the muscularis propria, and there is the development of elastosis in the teniae (Whiteway & Morson, 1985). There are also changes in the structure and function of the colon which are related to prolonged exposure to diets low in residue. These changes are slow in development and accumulate in the elderly. The relative contribution of the muscular changes with aging and the changes as a result of environmental influences remain matters of speculation. Since changes that are environmentally induced are preventable and possibly reversible with treatment, this relationship is a matter of intense ongoing interest.

Defecation

Changes in bowel habits, or the patterns of defecation, are foci for much concern of the elderly for their health. Constipation is of more frequent concern than diarrhea. Much of what passes for constipation really represents the patient's satisfaction or lack thereof with their bowel movements rather than ineffective, incomplete, or infrequent movements. Whether or not there is a problem of disturbed physiology, there is still a clinical management problem. Self-medication with laxatives adds additional possibilities for disturbance of normal defecation.

A standard for the normal frequency of bowel movements has not proven to be very helpful in the evaluation of individual patient problems. Interviews with healthy adults give a range of normal from three bowel movements daily to one movement a week. Most interviewees fell into the range of two movements per day to one movement every third day. A more useful clinical appraisal would address changes in regularity rather than the frequency of bowel movements per se. Unexplained irregularity warrants investigation. Understanding the normal physiology of defecation is essential to the orderly evaluation of the pathophysiology of abnormalities of bowel habit.

Our understanding of the sequence of events for normal defecation reveals only one change related to the aging of the rectum, stiffening of the rectal wall. The anal orifice is kept closed and sealed by the actions of three muscles—the internal sphincter, the external sphincter, and the puborectalis (Ihre, 1974)—and by an interdigitating plug of epithelium and underlying vascular tissue collectively called the anal cushions (Gibbons, et al., 1986). The study by Ihre is perhaps the best outline of the physiology of defecation and is the prime source for this summary.

The internal sphincter is a circular ribbon of thickened smooth muscle continuous with the circular muscle of the colon. Its steady state is tonic contraction. It contributes approximately 80 per cent of the force contracting the sphincter at rest. It surrounds the upper two thirds of the anal canal. The external sphincter is comprised of striated muscle and surrounds the lower two thirds of the anal canal. With the sphincter at rest, tonic contraction of this muscle provides about 20 per cent of the squeeze of the sphincter. The external sphincter is capable of additional voluntary or reflex contraction, which is referred to as phasic contraction as compared with tonic contraction. The puborectalis is a loop of striated muscle which shares innervation and response with the external sphincter. It surrounds the anal canal and the internal sphincter immediately above the external sphincter. It also has both tonic and phasic contraction. The action of this muscle not only adds to the sphincter squeeze but also draws the anorectal junction forward establishing an angle, the rectal angle, that facilitates the sealing of the anal opening.

Material enters the rectal ampulla from the sigmoid colon. Even small volumes, as little as 20 ml, will cause reflex relaxation of the internal sphincter with the integrity of the seal maintained by the tonic contraction of the puborectalis and the external sphincter. This permits the rectal contents to descend into the anal canal to the level at which feces can be distinguished from gas or fluids. The discrimination of solids from gas is excellent, but discrimination of liquids from gas is poor. With a small volume in the ampulla, the tone quickly returns to the internal sphincter. As the volume accumulating in the ampulla rises to about 25 per cent of the maximum capacity of the rectum, the individual senses the urge to defecate. Voluntary as well as reflex contraction of the external sphincter and the puborectalis compensates for the waning effectiveness of the internal sphincter maintaining continence as the ampulla distends. At a maximal filling volume and/ or pressure, the internal sphincter is completely relaxed, and when contraction of the external sphincter and the puborectalis is voluntarily inhibited, the anal canal opens to permit evacuation of the contents of the rectum and colon. This emptying may be facilitated by straining (increase of the intraabdominal pressure) and by squatting. Clinically larger volumes are more easily evacuated than smaller, and the softer the consistency of the feces the easier its passage through the anal canal.

Emptying of the ampulla initiates a closing reflex that restores the muscle tone to the sphincter and the rectal angle. The selective passing of flatus is facilitated by the generation of high pressures in the ampulla by straining without distention sufficient to completely relax the sphincter. The gas escapes, with the partially contracted sphincter retarding the passage of formed stool.

Ihre observed only one change with aging. The maximum tolerated volume in the rectum was smaller in elderly patients, while the maximum tolerated pressure remained unchanged. The maximal volumes observed averaged 400 ml in young adults and 320 ml in the elderly. A given volume in an elderly individual would produce a higher pressure than the identical volume in a younger individual. This suggests that the rectal wall stiffens with age.

REFERENCES

Gibbons, C.P., et al.: Role of anal cushions in maintaining continence. Lancet 1:886–888, 1986.

Ihre, T.: Studies on anal function in continent and incontinent patients. Scand J Gastroenterol 9:5–64, 1974.

Ritchie, J.A.: Colonic motor activity and bowel function. Gut 9:442, 502, 1971.

Whiteway, J., and Morson, B.C.: Elastosis in diverticular disease of the sigmoid colon. Gut 26:258–266, 1985.

Chapter 5
BOWEL HABIT
William A. Sodeman, Jr.

The perception that one's bowel function mirrors the state of one's general health is entrenched in folklore that must date to prehistory. In the not too distant past, the ravages of the various diarrhea and dysentery-producing infections associated with poor personal and public hygiene gave substance to the presumption of importance concerning the state of one's bowels.

For the last century there has been intermittent enthusiasm in scientific and medical circles for a more basic association between bowel function and health. With the identification of bacterial inhabitants in the colon and with the understanding of their role as direct and toxin-producing pathogens, the concept that sluggish bowels give rise to autointoxication by absorbed bacterial products has had a substantial vogue. Good scientific evidence to refute the autointoxication theories has not effectively displaced them from the public mind. Cleansing the colon of bacteria and toxins with daily laxatives and/or frequent enemas was very much a part of the growing-up process of many current members of the geriatric population.

There is ample recent emphasis that bulk, usually in the form of dietary fiber, has some benefit in the colon; the backlash from this has been a renewed interest by members of the geriatric population in frequent functioning bowels. However, the elderly often do not distinguish the difference between nonabsorbable bulk and other laxatives, purges, and enemas in regulating bowel habit. The result is a significant portion of the geriatric population with an unwarranted concern about bowel function. Hidden among them is a much smaller, yet not insignificant, group with diarrhea, constipation, incontinence, or change in bowel habit that is of real clinical significance. There is also a subset of this group that self-medicates to the point of laxative abuse.

Communication with the elderly concerning bowel habit takes patience largely in the definition of terms. There are no standard norms for bowel habit, although there are thresholds which, when exceeded, should prompt inquiry rather than diagnosis. Generally, if a patient reports fewer than three movements weekly, a serious inquiry should be made with regard to constipation. If a patient reports liquid stools or more than three movements daily, then inquiry concerning diarrhea is in order.

The step from inquiry to diagnosis focuses on identifying the patient's own customary pattern of bowel habit. The onset of acute diarrhea or acute constipation should be marked by a change in this customary pattern. The patient (one of a surprising number) who customarily defecates only once a week merits real evaluation if there is a sudden unexplained change to a single daily stool. A patient who ordinarily passes three loose stools daily and who abruptly changes to a single daily formed stool has become costive, and this also warrants explanation.

A second step, essential for the diagnosis of chronic constipation or chronic diarrhea, is to share the patient's definition of the terms constipation and diarrhea. Constipation seems to be a larger semantic problem. To most physicians, constipation implies a reduction in the frequency of defecation with perhaps some difficulty in passing the stool. Many patients equate constipation with a sense of urgency, with a feeling of incomplete emptying, with the passage of small (volume) stools, with irregular bowel habits, or with any combination of the above, regardless of frequency of defecation. There are semantic problems with the word diarrhea as well. To some patients it is frequent movements, to others loose stools, and many others mean only watery movements. Without sharing the patient's definition, the history is meaningless and diagnosis is almost hopeless.

CONSTIPATION

Constipation is broadly defined as any irregularity of bowel habit associated with slowing of the frequency of stools. It can be acute or chronic, constant or intermittent. Its importance to the patient's health is directly related to the cause, but it is wise to remember that even though the cause is trivial and without pathological significance, the problem may still require management for the well-being of the patient.

Constipation of Recent Onset

An acute change of bowel habit should be a trigger for prompt evaluation carried to the point of diagnosis. Acute problems can include life-threatening emergencies, and the pace of evaluation needs to reflect this. Constipation is an unusual presenting symptom for acute intestinal obstruction. Usually symptoms or signs related to the underlying obstruction or clinical manifestations proximal to the point of obstruction overshadow any change in daily bowel habit. Intermittent or partial obstruction can easily present as constipation.

A careful history and thorough physical examination are the best guides to any further work-up or evaluation. Care in the history taking can usually be equated with understanding what the patient means by constipation and what has been the time sequence of its development. If one fails to understand what the patient means at the outset, then the work-up may be needlessly confused. Table 5–1 lists the common causes of constipation.

Clinical Evaluation

When a patient presents with a primary complaint of constipation of recent onset, the first concern should be to establish some kind of time line for the development of the problem. This may not be as simple as it sounds. Most people in the United States have one or two bowel movements daily. A two-day lapse in the call to stool would not be unusual and, to most, not a cause for alarm. However, in some

TABLE 5–1. Common Causes of Constipation

Motility abnormality	Mechanical obstruction
Idiopathic pseudo-obstruction	Hernia: inguinal, femoral, internal
Acute exacerbation of diverticulosis	Volvulus: caecal, sigmoid
Dermatomyositis	Tumors
Myotonic dystrophy	Rectocele
Diabetic enteropathy	Adhesions
Vascular insufficiency	Fecal impaction
Metabolic abnormalities	**Diet**
Hypokalemia	Decreased intake
Diabetic acidosis	Decreased fiber
Hypothyroidism	Idiosyncratic reaction to specific foods
Hypercalcemia	**Drugs**
Uremia	Anticholinergics
Inflammation	Aluminum-containing antacids
Acute diverticulitis	Calcium-containing antacids
Fissure in ano	Iron
Fistula in ano	Opiates
Thrombosed hemorrhoid	**Idiopathic**
Inflammatory bowel disease	
Ulcerative proctitis	
Campylobacter proctitis	

patients it would be cause for panic. For an acute abdominal catastrophe to present as a primary complaint of constipation requires a patient who is hypersensitive to changes in bowel habit. Most of the time these hypersensitive patients have no intestinal disease, and the decision concerning recurrent evaluation with each episode becomes a real management problem. Fortunately, most patients will appreciate other signs and symptoms of an abdominal catastrophe long before they could appreciate slowing of the frequency of defecation. Patients who claim constipation and who have only a trivial fluctuation in bowel habit deserve protection from repeated evaluation. The conundrum is the timely identification of the patient in whom constipation means real disease.

Acute Constipation

A sudden onset of constipation which can be appreciated by the patient raises the spectre of abdominal emergency. Acute vascular insufficiency, incarceration in a hernia, sigmoid or cecal volvulus, and specific and nonspecific proctitis can all have an early presentation of acute constipation before the full expression of the clinical problem becomes evident. Physical findings of inflammation in the abdomen even though mild should trigger a complete blood count, measurement of serum electrolytes, a flat and upright abdominal x-ray, and consideration of a proctosigmoidoscopy. Should these prove nondiagnostic, one is faced with opting for expectant observation or angiography. An infrequently used but often very helpful intermediate step can be a four quadrant peritoneal tap searching for fluid and white cells that can offer objective evidence of intraabdominal inflammation.

If clinical findings or delays prior to seeking evaluation indicate that the problem is of recent but not acute onset, management of the diagnostic process can be stepwise and thoughtful.

Motility Abnormalities

Motility disturbances of many different etiologies can present as constipation of recent onset. Many of these do not have, to the patient at least, an obvious association with bowel function, and they must be dug out of the history with specific questioning. Examples include diabetes, hypokalemia, antiparkinsonian therapy, and oral iron therapy. At the very least a careful history can develop a working differential diagnosis, and often it will yield a specific cause for the constipation. Physical findings in motility disturbances tend to be a little bland unless you catch a patient with dermatomyositis or with idiopathic pseudo-obstruction during an attack. The absence of physical findings reassures that an acute emergency is unlikely but leaves one plodding on with more and more elaborate diagnostic maneuvers. Rectal examination and proctosigmoidoscopy add little to the diagnosis of a motility disorder. Management is essentially the management of the underlying motility problem. Unfortunately, the pathophysiology of most of these problems is so poorly understood that symptomatic treatment is all that can be offered.

Inflammation

Inflammation in the peritoneal cavity is likely to result in ileus. If the inflammation is focal and distal in the digestive tube, then the ileus may remain focal and distal, and constipation may be the presenting symptom. Early responses to inflammation in elderly patients can be muted without necessarily the leucocytosis, fever, and localizing pain that would be characteristic in a younger patient. Even minor evidence of intraabdominal inflammation is worthy of follow-up in this setting. Inflammatory bowel diseases—both Crohn's and chronic ulcerative colitis—may have the initial onset after age 65. Perianal inflammatory disease may be an additional sign of intraabdominal inflammation or may itself be responsible for constipation. Painful defecation as a result of a fissure, abscess, or fistula in ano or even a thrombosed hemorrhoid may inhibit defecation to the point of constipation. The resultant hard dry scybala worsen the problem with each successful passage. Fortunately, inspection and digital examination can provide rapid diagnosis as well as some relief and can indicate the direction for further assessment. Pain may limit the use of digital exam and may require preliminary treatment with topical anti-inflammatory agents and stool softeners as well as the use of topical anesthetics during the examination. General anesthesia is rarely required to permit adequate examination.

Inflammatory constipation is best managed by specific measures directed at the underlying inflammatory process. Often there is a need for symptomatic measures to restore the normal pattern of bowel habit.

Mechanical Obstruction

The most common cause of mechanical obstruction to bowel movements is a fecal impaction. Many other causes of partial or complete obstruction are found in the elderly, although only a few have a real predilection for this age group (Table 5–2). Obstruction by a tumor is an ever-present worry in the elderly patient, and volvulus (caecal, transverse colon, or sigmoid) is also a particular problem. All problems due to mechanical obstruction should convey a sense of urgency in management.

TABLE 5–2. Mechanical Obstruction as a Cause of Constipation

Fecal impaction	Inflammatory stricture
Tumor	Crohn's disease
Hernia	Diverticulitis
Inguinal	Postirradiation
Femoral	Adhesions
Internal	Endometriosis
Rectocele	Pseudo-obstruction
Volvulus	
Caecal	
Transverse colon	
Sigmoid	

Impaction

There are multiple mechanisms that can produce fecal impaction, and often several factors become additive in a patient. The elderly seem particularly susceptible to its development. These factors are listed in Table 5–3.

A decrease in dietary intake and a shift, which is sometimes voluntary and sometimes forced, to a bland dietary intake may deprive the patient of necessary cues that have heretofore been stimulants of regular bowel habits. A decrease in calorie intake has been regularly observed in the elderly (Kane, et al., 1984) and is in part due to a fall in the metabolic rate with aging. This fall in calorie intake often takes the form of irregular, small, or skipped meals. For many patients the loss of the breakfast stimulus for the gastrocolic reflex leads directly to irregular bowel habits. A bland and monotonous diet forced on some elderly by economic misfortune and on others by institutionalization only adds to this problem. The loss of bulk in the diet as a result of extensively processed and residue-free foods only exacerbates the decrease in overall calorie intake.

The mechanism by which physical activity stimulates bowel action is in no way clear, but the clinical observation of a relationship between inactivity and constipation and then impaction seems rock solid. Decrease in physical activity is a common but not necessary accompaniment of aging, and impaction is a frequent result. The effect that

TABLE 5–3. Common Causes of Fecal Impaction

Decreased dietary intake
Decreased dietary fiber
Decreased physical activity
Depression
Impaired sensation in the rectal vault
Poor access to toilet facilities
"Voluntary" constipation
Dementia—inattention to call to stool

depression has on bowel function is equally obscure but also real and adds to the problem of impaction in the elderly.

There are a number of patients who suffer a true decrease in sensation in the rectal vault. Often this is associated with a past history of laxative abuse, but the confusion associated with dementia can also be a factor. Many patients with decreased mobility find toilet facilities inconvenient or impossible to access on demand and therefore suppress the call to stool. A few patients reacting with hostility to caregivers withhold the "desirable" bowel movement to "get back" at the caregiver, a kind of voluntary constipation.

In all cases the end result is a rectal vault filled with desiccating stool. The large hard scybala that form cannot be passed mechanically despite the sense of urgency that they may induce. This continuous stimulus by unrelieved distention may result in loose stool flowing around the impacted feces, with the seeming paradox of diarrhea induced by impaction.

Digital examination will provide the diagnosis and often the opportunity for treatment if the impaction can be broken up with the gloved finger. Rectal administration of stool softeners is occasionally necessary. Equal in importance to resolution of the impaction is the prevention of its re-formation. This involves the provision of adequate bulk, attention to meal content, timely access to toilet facilities, exercise, and a host of other factors that must be matched to the patient's problems in order to be successful.

Mechanical obstruction other than impaction is usually a major medical problem. Colon cancer and volvulus are considered in detail further in this chapter. Although not necessarily a problem of the aged, obstruction by incarceration in hernias and as a result of rectoceles are also in the differential diagnosis of constipation of recent onset.

Diet

As outlined in the discussion of impaction, dietary factors play an important role in the maintenance of normal bowel habit. In spite of strong folk tradition, few if any foods provoke constipation, although there are many reports of idiosyncratic responses of individuals to specific foods. The absence of some food and nutritional components has a much stronger association with failing bowel function. Many foods, particularly fresh fruits and vegetables, contain natural laxative compounds (e.g., prunes and green apples), and a shift to a bland diet will result in sluggish bowel action. Often individuals have an idiosyncratic sensitivity to specific foods. In addition, many elderly people suffer from dietary changes when they move to live with friends or relatives or in and out of institutional care.

A second dietary feature that seems to play a role in the development of constipation is the deficit of nonabsorbable residue or bulk in the diet. Because the largest component of this nonabsorbable residue seems to be fiber, this is commonly called fiber deficiency. Careful examination of the literature will reveal a host of claims and refutations concerning both the need for fiber in the diet and the value of supplementation of the diet with bran in the treatment of various problems. Several points seem well established. Unrefined foods contain significantly more fiber than the highly refined foods found in Western society. Regardless of country of residence or social affiliation, stool bulk remains high in traditional unrefined diets. When individuals have a lifelong experience with a diet rich in fiber, they do not suffer many of the digestive tract and rectal conditions prevalent in our society. This includes appendicitis, diverticulosis, diverticulitis, hiatal hernia, inguinal hernia, and colon cancer. The epidemiological relationship seems soundly based. All of these problems can be associated with slow or difficult transit through the colon and/or difficult defecation. Yet most of the clinical difficulty occurs with the attempt to treat a variety of problems associated with transit or defecation by adding fiber to the diet.

The best working definition for dietary fiber seems to be ". . . a convenient term for the supporting structures for plant cell walls and substances intimately associated with them" or indigestible plant-derived foodstuffs (The Royal College of Physicians, 1980). Accordingly, under the umbrella term "fiber" one can include many diverse compounds and preparations in addition to cellulose. There are noncellulose carbohydrates, lignins, gums, and protein constituents. In addition, the composition of the fiber will vary among plant species, with the part of the plant selected, i.e., root, stem, leaf, or seed, and even with the degree of maturity of the plant. Therapeutic results are likely to be deeply influenced by the selection of the source for the fiber. At least some of the reported inconsistencies among studies of fiber therapy must relate to the possible variability in fiber composition.

In the management of constipation with fiber it is wise to gain familiarity with two preparations, bran and psyllium, as benchmarks against which the effectiveness and utility of other preparations can be measured. Bran is cheap and readily available in the supermarket, but many patients find it unpalatable or unacceptable. Psyllium is somewhat more expensive but is also an over-the-counter preparation and is formulated in a variety of highly palatable preparations. A significant number of patients are unprepared to accept bran, which to them represents food rather than medicine, yet are quite willing to accept psyllium formulated and sold as a drug. One needs at least this range of choices to get past the first therapeutic hurdle, the regular and consistent supplementation with fiber. There are patients who are unable, for a variety of reasons ranging from unpalatability to absence of teeth, to use coarse fiber supplements. There are alternative preparations in tablet form or in fiber-supplemented foods which can be used.

The therapeutic goal is the regular administration of enough fiber to result in the passage of one or two soft bowel movements daily. For reasons that are poorly understood, there is a great deal of individual variation from patient to patient in response to fiber. The amount and timing of the fiber supplement must be adjusted to the individual patient to achieve optimum results. Many patients request, and a few demand, a fiber diet rather than spoonsful of psyllium or bran. Our experience is that in patients who genuinely need supplementation, diet lacks the sensitivity in dose adjustment and frequently provides insufficient fiber to achieve optimum benefit unless it is carried to bizarre extremes. It is possible to overdose on fiber with bloating and flatulence as a result. A safe starting point is two teaspoonsful (heaping) of bran moistened in the mouth with a beverage of choice. Citrus juices seem to work well. The bran is chewed and swallowed and is followed by two full glasses of liquid. Psyllium is usually mixed with water or a beverage. Among untoward side effects described is bolus obstruction of the intestine by fiber that was inadequately diluted with fluid when taken. Additional adverse effects that may need to be considered include decreased absorption of iron and calcium, which occurs with fiber ingestion, and the possibility of precipitation of complete obstruction in the intestine at a site of subacute or incomplete obstruction. By using one or more spoonsful daily and by adjusting the administration to one or more times a day, the dosage becomes infinitely variable, and few patients will be found who cannot be regulated with bran or psyllium. This form of management does require patience on the part of the physician and the patient alike. Frustration and impatience in one or both parties are responsible for most of the incomplete or failed therapies with fiber.

Drugs

A wide variety of drugs can cause constipation. In few this is the primary drug effect, but more often constipation is an unsought-after side effect of the drug. A patient presenting with constipation of recent onset merits careful review of current medication history in an attempt to uncover a potential offender. A history of proprietary as well as prescription drugs should be elicited, or important clues will be overlooked. Drugs are frequent contributors to constipation of multifactorial etiology.

Opiates. Narcotic analgesics and their analogs were often used in the past in the control of acute and chronic diarrhea. The development of several new analogs with a primary action on the gastrointestinal tract and with little or no analgesic potential has largely eliminated the prescription of drugs with a high addictive potential as antidiarrheals. Opiate drugs are used in the management of both acute and chronic pain, and many patients fail to associate this therapy with an altered bowel habit.

Anticholinergics. Drugs with major anticholinergic effects are widely employed in the treatment of the elderly (Table 5–4). Many of the preparations used in the management of Parkinson's disease have their anticholinergic action as their prime effect on the central nervous system. A direct action on the intestine is a result, and side effects include both constipation and diarrhea. Similarly, a number of potent anticholinergics are employed in the management of urinary incontinence. These drugs, selected for their direct effect on the smooth muscle of the bladder, share an identical action on the smooth muscle of the intestine. The third broad category of drugs with anticholinergic effects are the antidepressants. With this group of drugs, the anticholinergic effects are not sought after, and a number of drugs varying in their anticholinergic potential have been marketed. These drugs can be characterized in terms of their anticholinergic effect in a spectrum from very high (e.g., amitriptyline) to very low (e.g., trazodone) and all

TABLE 5–4. Drugs with Anticholinergic Effects

Management of Parkinson's Disease
Trihexyphenidyl (Artane)
Benztropine (Cogentin)
Management of Incontinence
Propantheline (Pro-Banthine)
Oxybutynin (Ditropan)
Dicyclomine (Bentyl)
Flavoxate (Urispas)
Imipramine (Tofranil, SK-Pramine, Janimine)
Management of Depression
Tricyclic
    Amitriptyline (Elavil, Endep, Etrafon, Limbitrol, Triavil)
    Doxepin (Sinequan, Adapin)
    Imipramine (Tofranil, SK-Pramine, Janimine)
    Desipramine (Norpramin, Pertofrane)
    Protriptyline (Vivactil)
    Nortriptyline (Pamelor)
    Amoxapine (Asendin)
Tetracyclic
    Maprotiline (Ludiomil)
Other
    Trazodone (Desyrel)

Modified from tables in Kane, R. L., et al.: Essentials of Clinical Geriatrics. New York, McGraw-Hill, 1984.

gradations in between. There is a great deal of individual variation in sensitivity to anticholinergic effects with a few people being unusually sensitive and even fewer highly resistant. It is unusual to have constipation prove to be the limiting factor in the use of these drugs. The patient may be comforted by the addition of symptomatic measures to offset constipation at the first sign of its appearance.

Antacids. Aluminum and calcium-containing antacids are common culprits in the precipitation of constipation. Because they are readily available at candy counters and grocery store checkout lanes, they are easily overlooked by a patient when questioned concerning current medications. The problem is simply managed by the addition and/or substitution of a magnesium-containing antacid with a cathartic action. Often alternating antacids is necessary to keep the patient comfortable.

Management of constipation resulting from the other classes of drugs mentioned above may not be so simple. Often nonspecific measures to prevent or relieve the constipation are preferable to accepting a less adequate drug for the treatment of the primary problem.

Chronic Constipation

Most of the mechanisms responsible for constipation of acute onset are also the cause of chronic constipation. Diet, drugs, and motility abnormalities are the frequent offenders; and multiple factors are common. With constipation of recent onset, there is at least a reasonable likelihood that there will be an underlying factor that can be identified and treated. Without the significant features of recent historical change to guide the physician, the work-up of chronic constipation is far less rewarding. The balance between the meager yield, the cost of extensive work-up, and the gravity of missing tumor, vascular embarrassment, or other mechanical obstruction is not an easy one to arrive at, particularly in an elderly patient with other health problems. Many patients have established a longstanding peaceful coexistence with their chronic constipation; in fact if one carefully defines what the patient means by constipation, there may be no pathologic physiology at all. Often the patient's response to perceived constipation is a regimen of cathartics that itself leads to physiological difficulty; this practice needs to be modified or, if possible, stopped.

Irritable Bowel Syndrome

Among younger and middle-aged patients, irritable bowel syndrome is among the most common causes of constipation. In the aging patient, as other mechanisms for constipation become operative, the percentage ascribable to irritable bowel syndrome falls, although it continues to be a problem. Most studies find patients with irritable bowel syndrome to have normal to slow transit times (Ritchie, 1986) with significant slowing at the sigmoid colon (Misiewicz, 1975). There is some evidence of hyperactivity of the smooth muscle of the rectosigmoid (Chowdhury, et al., 1976). The result is the gradual release of small fecal pellets into the rectum. Among the few documented age-related changes in the rectum is a reduction of the volume required to stimulate the urge to defecate. These pellets are an effective stimulus. Recent studies (Bannister, et al., 1985) indicate that pellets in the rectum become increasingly difficult to expel as their diameter decreases below 2.5 cm. At a diameter of 0.5 cm, normal volunteers are unable to voluntarily expel the pellet. This scenario suggests that small pellets of stool (pellets capable of stimulating the urge to defecate but of a size too small to be evacuated without strain) are released through a hyperactive rectosigmoid segment.

Management of this sort of constipation is largely symptomatic. However, there is some evidence that the provision of bulking agents can relieve this sigmoid spasm (Manning, et al., 1977) and move the patient toward normal, comfortable bowel habits.

Neurological Constipation

Chronic constipation secondary to neurological mechanisms may be difficult to diagnose and is always a problem to manage. The distal colon is innervated with parasympathetic fibers from sacral segments that enter the colon through the pelvic nerve trunks. Destruction of these nerves results in a loss of sensation, intrinsic reflexes, and hypomotility and leaves the patient unable to defecate spontaneously. Low cord lesions interfere with the external anal sphincter as well. These are not problems of aging, although they can occur in the elderly. Changes associated with the neuropathy of diabetes mellitus can present as constipation as well as the more frequent complaint of diarrhea. Careful management of the diabetes permits time for an emergence of secondary complications in the elderly. A number of management options are available in this context (see Chapter 3).

Much more insidious are the less well-defined neuropsychological mechanisms that produce a rectum insensitive to distention with stool. These patients miss the call to stool eventually resulting in an impaction. Multiple mechanisms have been suggested ranging from organic neuropathy as an age change to simple inattention in patients with senile dementia. Environmental factors such as inaccessibility of toilet facilities and even rage directed at the caregiver may result in "voluntary" constipation. Management of these problems has been previously discussed in the section on impaction.

A subset of patients with incoordination of muscles of the pelvic floor during the act of defecation have been identified (Turnbull, et al., 1986). These individuals suffer a failure of the ability to expel a rectal bolus. Management with fiber or softeners is not effective; often these patients must resort to mechanical aids such as a rectal tube to evacuate the rectum.

Management of Constipation

Few health problems offer the patient the opportunity for self-management that constipation does. Pharmacies and supermarkets are replete with laxatives of all types and potencies. Television and the print media overflow with advertisements stressing the healthfulness of regularity and offering products to ensure this state. The elderly are a responsive audience. Therefore, management of constipation in the elderly is a two-part task that includes disengagement of the patient from inappropriate therapies and institution of safe and effective remedies.

In truth, all classes of laxatives and cathartics have some appropriate medical application, but for many the proper therapeutic opportunities are infrequent in occurrence. A partial list of laxatives by class is found in Table 5–5. Selection of the appropriate agent is another balancing act for which consideration must be given to the patient's physiological need, the mechanism of action of the drug, complicating conditions, and patient acceptance.

Fiber

Bulking agents are perhaps the most useful of all of the laxatives in the management of the constipated elderly patient. They have been

TABLE 5–5. Common Laxatives and Cathartics

Bulking Agents	**Saline Cathartics**
Bran	Magnesium sulfate (Epsom salts)
Psyllium	Magnesium hydroxide (milk of
Methylcellulose	magnesia)
Guyar gum	Sodium and potassium phosphate
Tragacanth	Citrate
Agar	Mineral waters (various)
Emollients	**Osmotic Agents**
Dioctyl sodium sulfosuccinate	Lactulose
Mineral oil	Sorbitol
Stimulants	Lactose
Phenothalin	**Rectal Agents**
Cascara sagrada	Bisacodyl
Senna	Glycerin
Castor Oil	Carbon dioxide
Bisacodyl	Soap suds
Danthron	Saline solution
	Sodium or potassium phosphate
	Water

with us since the very beginnings of medical history. The writings of Hippocrates in the fifth century BC include, "Wholemeal bread cleans out the gut and passes through as excrement. White bread is more nutritious as it makes less faeces" (The Royal College of Physicians, 1980). The fortunes of bulking agents over the centuries have been linked with their value as foodstuffs rather than as medicinals. It is only recently that their physiological role in the health of the bowel has come to receive much attention.

Bulking agents generally are considered to be equivalent to dietary fiber. As mentioned earlier, these include a highly variable mixture of plant-derived compounds that share the property of being indigestible in the human (and mammalian) digestive tract. Ruminants provide for digestive tract storage of dietary fiber to permit bacterial action to reduce the fiber to digestible molecules. A few nonruminants, including leaf-eating monkeys and hamsters, provide for nonrumen storage in the digestive tract to permit necessary bacterial action.

Mammalian digestive tracts are equipped to digest alpha glycans which include starch and glycogen. The remaining plant polysaccharides include beta glycans (cellulose and other beta glycans) and heteroglycans. Heteroglycans include pectins, hemicelluloses, gums, and algal polysaccharides such as agar. The only noncarbohydrate components of dietary fiber are the lignins. This is less esoteric than it at first sounds, since a number of compounds are marketed as dietary fiber even though they may be less effective in the digestive tract as bulking agents. While many of these agents, pectins and gums particularly, do have application in the management of constipation, it seems wise to rely on bran and psyllium. Both are high in cellulose and are excellent bulk producers in the digestive tract.

Psyllium preparations are derived from the plantago seed, a variety of plantain. The preparation contains cellulose as well as a variety of mucilaginous gums. It is an excellent bulk former, and the gums may contribute to the reduction in serum cholesterol by binding bile acids in gut lumen. The many commercial formulations vary in the amount of absorbable carbohydrate added, usually to improve taste, and in the amount of sodium. By careful selection one can find formulations acceptable to diabetics and patients with cardiovascular disease. They are marketed in a wide variety of easily mixed palatable forms that allow for the dose adjustment required to get optimal benefit. Careful attention must be paid to ensure that these and any bulking agents are taken with adequate oral fluids. Intestinal obstruction by a bolus of bulking agent, in some cases resulting in death, has been reported. These occurred in individuals with no organic obstruction lesion in the intestine (Souter, 1965). If bulking agents are carefully mixed with adequate amounts of liquid, they should pose no threat.

Bran is also available in many formulations. Coarse-milled bran provides more bulk per gram than any of the fine-milled or cereal preparations. It is important to realize that equal doses of bran in differing formulations are not interchangeable in terms of bulking effect. Dose adjustment has been discussed above. The goal is to produce one or two soft bowel movements daily. This requires patience and individual adjustment of the dose for each patient.

Bulking agents are contraindicated in patients with mechanical obstruction and must be used with caution in patients with active colitis. Their use is also guarded in patients with acute and chronic intestinal vascular insufficiency which often simulates a mechanical obstruction because of the associated ileus. They are not helpful in patients with neuromuscular disease resulting in ileus. A few patients who have a rapid transit time respond to bulking agents with a slowing of transit; however, these patients are rarely constipated. Most other varieties of constipation will be benefited by therapy with a bulking agent. Preparations must be taken with enough oral fluid to prevent the formation of a bolus.

Emollients

Emollient agents include mineral oil and dioctyl sulfosuccinates. Mineral oil is an indigestible petroleum derivative with a very limited absorption by the human intestine. Its primary use is as a stool softener. Its action is slow in onset, usually requiring one to three days to have an effect. Chronic use is associated with some interference with the absorption of lipid-soluble vitamins. Patients with even minor, subclinical, swallowing function abnormalities may have trouble with this heavy oil and may aspirate, with the subsequent production of lipid granulomas in the lung. Mineral oil is readily available and is an historically popular laxative, although there is currently little indication for its use since more effective stool softeners are available. Occasional use by the patient who demands it is probably not harmful.

Dioctyl sulfosuccinates include sodium, calcium, and potassium salts. They all have a detergent-like effect and act as stool softeners. They do have a direct effect on mucosal salt and water absorption. Side effects are few in proper doses, but some drug interactions do occur with enhancement of the absorption. The primary use is to soften stools and to prevent straining at the time of defecation. This is desirable in patients with a recent myocardial infarction and following some kinds of surgery. Bulking agents will do a more effective job, but where patient preference or clinical circumstances dictate, the dioctyl sulfosuccinates have a place. They require one to three days to have an effect, depending on intestinal transit times.

Stimulants

Stimulant laxatives encompass three major groups. The diphenyl-amines include phenolphthalein and bisacodyl. They are modestly prompt in action, usually working in six to eight hours, and are effective as bedtime laxatives. They stimulate a formed stool rather than diarrhea. Bisacodyl has largely replaced phenolphthalein, although the latter remains available in some over-the-counter laxatives. The effective dose does vary from patient to patient, and it requires some adjustment. The primary use for bisacodyl is in the preparation of the bowel for x-ray or endoscopic procedures. It is an effective agent to use in the patient with acute constipation requiring short-term administration of a laxative while dietary and other adjustments are being made.

The anthracene group includes cascara sagrada, senna, and danthron. These are usually effective in a six- to eight-hour period and are not diarrhea producers. These drugs are commonly used as ingredients in over-the-counter laxatives; they are commonly associated with laxative abuse and related syndromes of electrolyte depletion. Chronic use results in the development of melanosis coli, which can be used as a marker to identify the potential laxative abuser. Although these drugs are acceptable for occasional use in the treatment of acute constipation, they may not be a wise choice in the management of chronic problems.

Castor oil is pressed from the seeds of *Ricinus communis*. The oil is hydrolyzed in the gut to produce ricinoleic acid which is the active principle. This is a powerful laxative with a rapid action—it usually produces watery diarrhea within one to three hours. Its only real use was in the preparation of the bowel for contrast x-ray, and it has largely been supplanted by milder preparations using saline cathartics and bisacodyl. In the rare case in whom a powerful purge is needed, this might be selected.

Saline Cathartics

Saline cathartics encompass a number of salts traditionally used to purge the intestine. Magnesium salts, including sulfate (Epsom salt), hydroxide (milk of magnesia), and citrate, are fast effective purges producing watery diarrhea in one to three hours. These salts share with other saline cathartics the mechanism of drawing water into the lumen to produce an isosmotic bolus that washes down the intestine. These can be effective laxatives when used in modest dosages. Milk of magnesia is the preferred form. Magnesium salts may utilize an alternate pathway by stimulating the release of cholecystokinin from the duodenal mucosa. This hormone has powerful motility effects on the distal colon, and its hormonal pathway would explain the prompt response noted in some patients. All of the saline cathartics are contraindicated in patients with renal insufficiency and in patients with cardiovascular disease who would be adversely affected by a sodium salt load or dehydration. The use of these salts as a purge in preparation for x-ray studies has been supplanted by milder regimens. As a laxative for relief of temporary constipation, magnesium hydroxide is the traditional favorite.

Sodium phosphate is a pleasant-tasting, rapid, effective cathartic that has gained wide acceptance as the preparation of choice before x-ray studies. Other saline mixtures with added polyethylene glycol have come into use in the preparation of patients for colonoscopy. These are isotonic mixtures of sodium chloride, sodium bicarbonate, sodium sulfate, and potassium chloride which, with the polyethylene glycol, provide a bolus to cleanse the gut without either dehydration or electrolyte absorption. The only real contraindications are obstruction, perforation, and active toxic colitis. In its use the patient's tolerance often turns out to be the limiting factor.

Mineral waters, most containing salts discussed above, have been employed for their laxative effects since prehistory. They occasionally offer an acceptable palatable alternative in patient management.

Osmotic Agents

Osmotic agents include all of the saline cathartics and several carbohydrate compounds as well. Sorbitol is a natural compound found in fruits, algae, and molasses. It has wide use as a sugar substitute particularly, in candies, and is a not infrequent cause of unexplained diarrhea in the calorie conscious. It is metabolized by some bacteria in the gut, but only slowly. Its prime use has been to cleanse the bowel of the patient with portosystemic enteropathy.

Lactulose is a synthetic dissacharide that is not digested in the small intestine and passes into the colon where it is fermented by the bacterial flora. In the small intestine the sugar exerts an osmotic effect, drawing a bolus of water into the lumen and purging the intestine. In the colon bacterial fermentation produces lactic and other acids which may also have an effect on colonic transit. The drug is principally used in the management of patients with portosystemic encephalopathy in whose guts ammonia is trapped. Its laxative effect has been helpful in the management of some patients with chronic constipation in whom the use of bulking agents has failed. It is slow in onset.

Lactose, the dissacharide of milk, may serve as an effective cathartic in patients who have congenital or acquired deficiency of lactase. In these patients the effect of lactose is essentially that of lactulose.

Rectal Agents

The contact action of bisacodyl is evident with rectal administration in either suppository or enema. The exact mechanism of production of a stimulus to defecate is not clear. Because of its rapid, reliable effect and the ease of administration, it is a popular adjunct to the preparation for x-ray and sigmoidoscopy. For the same reasons it is useful in the management of the patient who needs relief from acute constipation but who, for whatever reason, resists oral agents.

Glycerin as a suppository absorbs water and acts as a bolus stimulus to stimulate defecation. It is an old preparation and readily available. It receives much use in the management of patients with high spinal cord lesions. In addition, CO_2 is available in a suppository form, and it also acts as a bolus to initiate the defecatory urge. The suppository is moistened, then inserted, and it will slowly produce carbon dioxide. Within 10 to 20 minutes, enough distention to initiate defecation will occur. This too is often used in the management of patients with cord lesions.

Sodium phosphate enemas are available in convenient yet effective small-dose forms. These receive much use in preparation of the sigmoid for various procedures. They are also handy and useful for the patient who requires relief from acute constipation and who desires an enema. This has largely replaced the time-honored soap suds enema. Mineral oil is available in a small retention enema to provide stool softening in patients with recurrent impaction.

Laxative Abuse

Dependency

There is a voluntary component to the act of defecation which can be the focus of some change with aging. For many people the timing of bowel movements becomes regulated and highly specific. Environmental changes that interfere with established habit, such as travel, may result in much mental anguish and can be the cause of temporary constipation. Patients who are regular laxative users incorporate the laxative use into their bowel habit. What results is a dependency on laxatives to maintain regularity. Such a dependency in and of itself is not harmful. The long-term use of bulking agents is advocated but only in the sense of replacing fiber missing from the "normal" human diet. Chronic use of cathartics does set the stage for the development of complications associated with the use of some of these preparations.

Patients who have a loss of short-term memory may dose themselves with laxative, forget, and dose themselves again and again. This is an acute form of laxative abuse.

Melanosis coli is a condition of pigmentation of the colonic mucosa. It develops as a result of chronic ingestion of anthracene laxatives. Cascara is the most common offender. The pigmentation may involve the entire colon, but more often it is localized to the cecum and the rectum, the areas of stasis. It requires four to twelve months of chronic laxative use for development and will gradually fade with cessation of the laxatives. The mucosa rarely returns completely to normal. The condition appears to be benign, but it does serve as a marker for chronic laxative use which can be helpful in diagnosis.

Cathartic colon is a radiological diagnosis. With the chronic use of laxatives for 15 to 20 years, the colon acquires an appearance on barium enema which suggests chronic inflammatory disease. There is shortening and loss of haustration. The differentiation from inflammatory bowel disease is easily made by sigmoidoscopy. The muscosa appears normal without the friability and ulceration associated with colitis. The associated symptomatology is nonspecific and is more likely associated with the underlying problem that prompted chronic laxative administration in the first place. All of the classes of laxatives except the bulking agents have been implicated, but the irritant, stimulant laxatives seem to be the most common offenders. The appearance of the colon on x-ray will revert toward normal with cessation of the laxative use. Success in management is associated with success in controlling the underlying constipation.

In a few patients with chronic laxative use there will be significant electrolyte depletion, particularly of potassium. These patients will experience bouts of muscular weakness and dehydration. Although these respond promptly to potassium administration, they will reoccur. These patients seem to have an unusual sensitivity to diarrhea with rapid recurrence of weakness. It is thought that the chronic laxative use in these cases has damaged the mucosa making it susceptible to even minor stimuli.

Surreptitious or Inadvertent Laxative Abuse

The literature is replete with reports of factitial diarrhea in patients who are abusing laxatives but deny it when questioned. This minor variant of a Munchausen syndrome is usually an indicator of a significant emotional problem. It is important in the elderly that such neurotic or psychotic behavior be differentiated from simple confusion and from the inadvertent ingestion of laxatives in another guise, for example, in magnesium-containing antacids. In many patients these antacids produce an extraordinary laxative effect. Not all patients make the association between the administration of the antacids and the onset of the loose stools.

There are a number of laxative compounds which have become incorporated in processed foods and can lead to diarrhea that is clinically a mystery. Sorbitol is a common offender. This osmotic cathartic has wide use in the preparation of sugar-free chewing gum and candies. Many of these have moved from the dietetic shelf to the checkout lanes in the supermarket in an attempt to attract the calorie-conscious dieter. Diarrhea is an unexpected result. Fructose, a commonly employed sweetener in carbonated drinks, is incompletely absorbed and, when consumed in the heroic volumes sold by fast food outlets, can precipitate diarrhea that in fact represents laxative abuse.

DIARRHEA

The normal range of bowel habit extends to include a frequency of bowel movements which many individuals would label diarrhea. There is no genuinely satisfactory definition for diarrhea, and there are at least three independent variables—stool frequency, stool consistency, and the feeling of urgency. A single watery stool would properly be described with diarrhea, while far more frequent formed stools daily might evoke little concern. Many patients equate urgency without any change in stool consistency as diarrhea. As with constipation the most important feature is to share in the patient's definition of his or her normal bowel habit. Specific questions in the history will often be necessary to identify some patients who are suggestively abnormal. One needs to identify the frequency of bowel movements, their regularity, and their consistency. As with constipation the most significant feature is the occurrence of any change from the normal habit. Table 5–6 outlines the broad categories of causes of diarrhea. Evaluation of acute and chronic diarrhea is treated in both the foregoing and following chapters under various specific headings.

Incontinence

Few things are as disabling to a patient as fecal incontinence. While it is an uncommon problem in the young, it is a frequent occurrence in the aged. Incontinence should always prompt a search for a treatable

TABLE 5–6. Categories of Diarrhea

Infection	Toxins and irritants
Viral	Idiosyncratic reactions to food
Bacterial	Bacterial toxins
Fungal	Bile salts
Protozoan	Laxative abuse
Helminth	Malabsorption
Metabolic	Vascular insufficiency
Hormonal	Impaction
Motility disturbances	Inflammatory bowel disease
	Idiopathic

etiology. While symptomatic measures are often the only management option, it is especially gratifying to find a treatable lesion that restores continence. Problems with fecal incontinence fall into four broad categories—colonorectal problems, neurological problems, fecal impaction, and laxative abuse.

Fecal incontinence may be an acute occurrence or it may become an established chronic problem. At its first appearance every effort should be made to identify the mechanism and to implement whatever changes are required to restore acceptable control. Failure to do this carries a substantial risk that the incontinence will become an established permanent feature. Few things can be as devastating to the quality of life as loss of bowel control. It often marks the end of home care and the beginning of nursing home placement. All epidemiological studies of the effect of nursing home placement suggest that it represents, for many patients, the quickening of the downhill spiral of deterioration.

Colonorectal Lesions

A number of colonorectal lesions are associated with incontinence; these are listed in Table 5–7 and are discussed below.

Perianal Disease. Perianal disease that damages or destroys sphincteric function has no specific predilection for the elderly, but with the prolongation of life there is a steady increase in the number of patients with these problems. The problem can be simple thrombosis or other hemorrhoidal inflammation or the more serious problems of fissure, fistula, or abscess. All of these problems are associated with constipation as well as incontinence—seemingly polar opposites. If pain predominates with spasm in the rectum and sphincter, then constipation is likely. If irritation is the primary feature, the incontinence will be a result. Mixtures can produce confusing patterns of symptomatology. If the perianal disease begins to extend into the sphincter, then the damage can weaken and impair function directly.

Essential to the management is control of the inflammatory process.

TABLE 5–7. Colonorectal Lesions and Incontinence

Perianal disease	Carcinoma of the rectum
Inflamed hemorrhoids	Autonomic neuropathy
Fistula in ano	Diarrhea of any cause
Fissure in ano	Prolapse of the rectum
Rectal abscess	Impaction
Posthemorroidectomy	
Proctitis	
Infectious	
Ulcerative	
Factical	

Often the limitation of damage will require some surgical intervention for incision and drainage. Surgery in the perianal region in the elderly requires special justification and planning. When a certain degree of alteration of bowel habit already exists either because of neuropathy or desensitization resulting from a prolonged laxative habit, then the outcome with restoration of continence following surgical intervention is less assured. There is some suggestion (Gibbons, 1986) that the vascular cushions that enlarge to form hemorrhoids in normal circumstances serve as vascular plugs, sensitive to straining, that aid in preservation of continence. Hasty removal of inflamed but treatable tissue may lead to a poor outcome.

Proctitis. Proctitis is also responsible for both constipation and incontinence. With proctitis there is the added factor that the irritation may prompt an outpouring of mucus adding to the frequency and the volume of the incontinence. If the problem is infectious, specific antimicrobial therapy is in order. *Campylobacter* infections are emerging as a frequent cause at all ages. Inflammatory bowel disease, as discussed elsewhere, does have its initial onset in the elderly in a significant number of cases. Irritation by a finger or instrument cannot be overlooked in the elderly; many have a fixation on regularity and will resort to digital or other assistance to promote a bowel movement. Repeated enemas, either saline or soap suds, may provoke serious irritation. The patient's desire to keep "cleaned out" in order to prevent embarrassing episodes of incontinence promotes a vicious cycle of enema, irritation, and incontinence.

Management rests with removing the irritation by appropriate intervention with specific agents and by breaking the cycle of enema or cathartic use. The ease and acceptability of flexible proctosigmoidoscopy even in the frail patient has greatly facilitated the management of all forms of incontinence.

Tumors. Carcinoma of the rectum can produce incontinence by several mechanisms acting alone or in concert. The mass itself may be a partial obstruction and irritant, with resulting small volumes of stool and mucus that are passed inadvertently. Infiltration by the tumor may damage nervous control or the sphincter directly. Diagnosis is usually within reach of the gloved finger.

Neuropathy. Autonomic neuropathy rarely presents as incontinence in the absence of other signs and symptoms that will lead to diagnosis. Diabetes is the most common offender in the elderly. Reference should be made to the discussion of autonomic neuropathy in Chapter 3.

Diarrhea. Any form of diarrhea if virulent enough can stress the sphincter to the point of incontinence. Most of the age-related changes in the rectum as well as the acquired problems reduce the threshold for sphincter failure in the elderly.

Rectal Prolapse. Prolapse is a problem particularly in older women. Mechanisms will be discussed in a later chapter. As the mucosa slides lower in the anal canal, it distorts normal sphincteric function. Increasing degrees of prolapse incrementally degrade the ability of the sphincter to remain continent in the face of stress.

Impaction. Impaction, as outlined above, is commonly associated with constipation in the elderly. The hard fecal mass serves as a stimulant to defecation but prevents actual passage of the fecal mass through the sphincter. Small amounts of fecal material and mucus as a result of the irritation will pass the impacted mass, and their inadvertent passage provides many episodes of incontinence. In the sedentary patient, regular rectal examination may be required to ensure freedom from this problem.

Neurological problems

Patients with lesions of the pelvic nerves or the spinal cord often become incontinent. If sensation is lost, continence is managed by regular cleansing of the lower bowel. If there is interference with sphincter function and loss of integrity, management can become difficult to impossible. Often it is possible to identify the rhythm of rectal filling for the individual patient. This permits timely intervention with a suppository to stimulate the evacuation of the filled rectum.

Patients with dementia may simply forget or be unresponsive to the call to stool. The magnitude of the problem varies with the degree of the dementia. Often it just takes a regular reminder by a thoughtful caregiver to keep the patient continent. In severely demented patients requiring nursing home placement, it is possible to utilize antidiarrheal medications with periodic evacuation of the rectum stimulated by enema or suppository. This form of management is easily susceptible to abuse and must be undertaken only within the context of skilled nursing care.

Laxative abuse

One manifestation of laxative abuse is the development of incontinence. Success in diagnosis is akin to skilled detective work. A return to continence is almost always possible if the patient is willing and cooperative and has the insight to follow a program to interrupt the laxative habit. Reference is made to the discussion of laxative abuse earlier in this chapter. A special problem may occur with preparation of elderly patients for radiological or endoscopic procedures. A preparative regimen that is readily tolerated by a younger patient may stress the older rectum resulting in incontinence. Warning the patient may at least relieve some of the anxiety should this occur. This is not laxative abuse, rather it is a laxative side effect. Another side effect is the leakage of mineral oil through the sphincter, which is often reported with the use of this laxative.

When specific avenues for management of incontinence are exhausted, there still remains some approaches to assist in the nursing care. The approach varies with the ability of the patients to understand their plight and to cooperate. A patient who is aware of the incontinence and is distressed and embarrassed by it can be helped to a program of control by retraining to a new pattern of bowel habit. A patient who is aware of the incontinence but indifferent to it requires an avenue of management different from the patient who remains unaware of the problem. Habit training with the assistance of an occasional small enema or suppository is only feasible in the cooperative, understanding patient. It is largely a matter of evoking confidence in a plan to restore a dependable pattern of bowel habits. It is a time-consuming process with no rapid avenue to results.

If the patient lacks the ability to understand and to cooperate, the state of continence becomes reduced to a nursing problem. Nursing care can be eased by careful management of diet to provide a steady volume of fiber and to avoid diarrheogenic foods. As mentioned above, there is the opportunity to use antidiarrheals interspersed with small enemas or suppositories to produce a regularity that permits nursing care to provide continence. Such a regimen demands the attention of nurses and physicians since it substitutes pharmacology for physiology. There is small room for error and none for neglect.

REFERENCES

Bannister, J.J., et al.: Experimental support for a simple model of defecation. Gut 26:A1131, 1985.

Chowdhury, A.R., et al.: Characterization of a hyperactive segment at the rectosigmoid junction. Gastroenterology 71:584–588, 1976.

Gibbons, C.P., et al.: Role of anal cushions in maintaining continence. Lancet 1:886–887, 1986.

Kane, R.L., et al. Essentials of Clinical Geriatrics. New York, McGraw-Hill, 1984.

Manning, A.P., et al.: Wheat fibre and irritable bowel syndrome. A controlled trial. Lancet 2:417–418, 1977.

Misiewicz, J.J.: Colonic motility. Gut 16:311–314, 1975.

Ritchie, J.A.: Colonic motor activity and bowel function. Part II: Distribution and incidence of motor activity at rest and after food and carbacol. Gut 9:502–511, 1986.

The Royal College of Physicians: Medical Aspects of Dietary Fibre. Turnbridge Wells, Kent, Pitman Medical, 1980.

Souter, W.A.: Bolus obstruction of gut after use of hydrophilic colloid laxatives. Br Med J 1:166–168, 1965.

Turnbull, C.K., et al.: Failure of rectal expulsion as a cause of constipation: Why fibre and laxatives sometimes fail. Lancet 1:767–769, 1986.

Chapter 6

DISEASES OF THE AGING COLON

William A. Sodeman, Jr.

DIVERTICULOSIS (SIGMOID OR LEFT-SIDED DIVERTICULOSIS)

Simple, uncomplicated diverticulosis is very rare in the young but steadily increases in prevalence with age. Environmental factors are fundamental determinants for the development of colonic diverticula, and the disease is absent in societies that maintain a fiber rich diet high in unprocessed foods. The generally accepted working estimate is that 50 per cent of the elderly in Europe and North America have diverticular disease (Thompson & Patel, 1986). Considerable controversy exists over the role that strictly age-related changes in the colon may play in the development of diverticula as contrasted with purely environmental factors that simply accumulate to produce an unusual prevalence in the aged. In any event, the management of the complications of diverticular disease focuses on the geriatric population.

Clinical Presentation

Uncomplicated diverticulosis is a clinically silent disease. The diverticula themselves cause neither alteration in normal colonic function nor production of signs or symptoms of abnormality. Uncomplicated diverticula cause no pain, no bleeding, no diarrhea, and no constipation. Because diverticula are so very common, there are many individuals with colonic diverticula who also have symptoms of functional bowel upset. The extent of this overlap has been large enough to stimulate the opinion that irritable bowel syndrome is an antecedent in the development of diverticulosis. This topic has been reviewed in detail by Thompson and Patel (1986), and I will summarize their conclusions.

Virtually the only evidence favoring a causal relationship between irritable bowel syndrome and diverticulosis is the common coincidence of the two syndromes. However, the popular estimate is that about 50 per cent of the elderly in the United States have diverticula, and 30 per cent have a history of irritable bowel syndrome. One would expect that by chance alone 50 per cent of irritable bowel patients would develop diverticula and 30 per cent of patients found with diverticula would have a history of irritable bowel syndrome. Barium enema, the diagnostic test for diverticulosis, is more likely to be performed on patients with lower bowel symptoms. Since most of the 50 per cent with diverticula alone have a disease that is clinically silent (undiscovered), the apparent coincidence of the two syndromes would appear even higher. A number of investigators (Weinreich & Andersen 1976; Ritchie, 1977) utilizing various stimuli have demonstrated that asymptomatic patients with diverticula had motility responses in the colon similar to normal patients, while patients with diverticula and nonspecific lower gastrointestinal complaints (pain, distention and irregularity) had the motility responses of patients with irritable bowel syndrome. Clearly the question concerning a causal relationship between the two syndromes is still unresolved, and at this time they are best treated as separate entities.

Pathology and Pathologic Physiology

Diverticula are thin-walled sacs of mucosa penetrating through the muscular coats of the colon. While they may be located at any level of the colon, most are concentrated in the sigmoid and in the descending colon. Their location around the circumference of the colon wall is highly specific. They occur at the points of penetration of the muscular coat by nutrient arteries. These points of penetration are on either side and adjacent to the mesenteric taenia and on the mesenteric side and adjacent to the antimesenteric taeniae. In a patient with many diverticula, these will be found lined up in rows running the length of the affected colon segment (Fig. 6–1). This localization places the diverticula in close relationship with the nutrient arteries and their accompanying veins. Around the mouth of the diverticulum there is concentrated a rich capillary bed (Figs. 6–2 and 6–3). This relationship is an important feature in the pathogenesis of bleeding diverticula. These are false or pseudo diverticula, and, unlike congenital diverticula, they lack the support of the muscular coats of the colon.

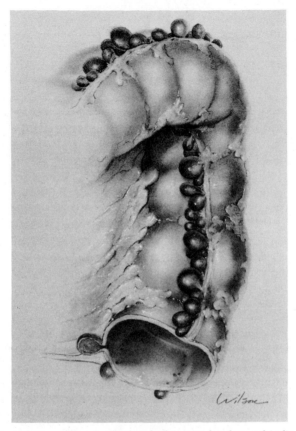

Figure 6-1. In patients with many diverticula they may be observed in lines adjacent to the two antimesenteric taeniae and adjacent to the mesenteric taenia.

Mendeloff (1986) has proposed a classification of types of diverticular disease of the colon (Table 6-1) which provides a useful outline for the consideration of the pathologic physiology of the disease(s). It seems likely on epidemiological and clinical grounds that diverticula limited to the right colon, solitary diverticulum, and simple massed diverticulosis each have a distinct pathogenic mechanism, and that these differ significantly from sigmoid diverticulosis. The final common path for all acquired diverticular disease is the formation of a closed chamber in the colon with an internal pressure adequate to cause a herniation of the mucosal lining of the colon through a weak spot in the colon wall. Part of the varied pathogenesis of the several colonic diverticular syndromes may rest with the nature of the weak spot. It seems likely that the definition of the closed chamber, the stimulus for the development of a critical pressure, and the nature of the weakness in the colon wall all may vary with each type of diverticular disease.

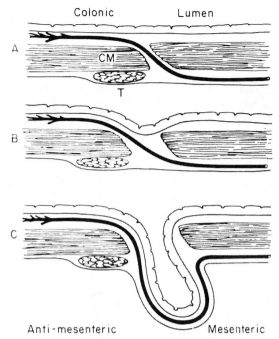

Colonic   Lumen

Anti-mesenteric   Mesenteric

Figure 6–2. Diverticula form in a constant relationship with the colon vascular supply. The protrusion of the mucosa is at a point of weakness in the circular muscle as a result of the penetration of the nutrient artery. The artery is lifted to ride over the dome of the diverticulum. Circular muscle (CM), taenia (T). (Reproduced with permission from Meyers, M. A., et al.: Pathogenesis of bleeding colonic diverticulosis. Gastroenterology 71:578, 1976. © by Williams & Wilkins 1976).

Aging of the colon muscle is accompanied by the development of elastosis in the taenia coli (Whiteway & Morson, 1985). The taenia function to provide structural integrity for the colon during motility events. Contraction of the taenia in a segment of colon with attendant increase in tension in the muscle stiffens the taenia and, in effect, results in a structural skeleton for circular muscle contraction. The colon contents also serve to stabilize the colonic segment. In the sigmoid these are formed elements capable of offering some resistance. To achieve requisite tensions, contractions of the taenia of a filled colonic segment need be much smaller than in an empty or near empty segment.

In addition, contractions of taenia will produce shortening of the segment. In a near empty segment, this will be profound, with collapse and compression of the colonic segment producing enhancement of muscular and mucosal folds at the expense of the lumen, much as the lumen narrows in a bunched-up sleeve in a sweater. This appearance of the colon was well described by Keith as early as 1910. Whiteway

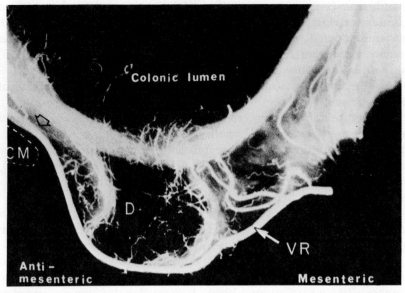

Figure 6–3. A radiograph of an injected specimen of colon containing a diverticulum (D). The position of the circular muscle (CM) is indicated by the open arrow. The angioarchitecture is well demonstrated with the rich capillary bed at the opening of the diverticulum and the vas rectum (VR) arching over the dome of the diverticulum. Compare this with Figure 6–2. (Reproduced with permission from Meyers, M. A., et al.: Pathogenesis of bleeding colonic diverticulum. Gastroenterology 71:578, 1976. © by Williams & Wilkins 1976).

TABLE 6–1. Types of Diverticular Disease of the Colon

Prediverticulosis
    Elastosis of taeniae coli
    Myochosis (thickened circular-muscle layer)
    Diverticula still in bowel wall, not protruding
Diverticulosis, multiple (? greater than two)
    Simple massed diverticulosis
    Diverticulosis of the right colon
    Diverticulosis of the left colon and/or sigmoid
        With spasm
        With history of irritable bowel syndrome
Diverticulosis, solitary
    Of the right colon and/or cecum
    Of the sigmoid, giant type
Diverticulitis
    With local inflammation
    With generalized peritonitis and/or perforation
    With penetration into adjacent structures; fistula formation
Generalized diverticulosis of small and large intestine

From Mendeloff, A. I.: Thoughts on the epidemiology of diverticular disease. Clin Gastroenterol 15:857, 1972. Reprinted with permission.

and Morson (1985) suggest that such shortening, when chronic, is a stimulus for elastosis, which in turn stabilizes the taenia and fixes the shortened pleated segment of colon. Effective treatment of diverticular disease by transverse taeniomyotomy as described by Hodgson (1973) lends support to this pathogenic mechanism.

As the colonic segment is compressed in length, the fasciculi of circular muscle narrow and crowd in on one another to produce a thickened muscular layer referred to as myochosis. Initially, this morbid anatomy was interpreted as hypertrophy of the circular muscle producing the thickening and rigidity, but light and electron microscopy studies of affected muscle reported by Whiteway and Morson (1985) reveal none of the cytological characteristics of hypertrophy. It is simply normal muscle bunched up together.

The pleating and overlapping of folds facilitate the formation of closed chambers during motility events. Further increase in tension in the wall of the closed chamber results in remarkable pressure increase in the lumen. This pressure is governed by the laws of Young and Laplace; thus, it depends on the ratio of wall tension to radius of the chamber ($P = kT/R$) (Guyton, 1986). The smaller the average chamber radius, the greater is the pressure for any given change in wall tension. This is an additional explanation of the prevalence of diverticula in the sigmoid, the narrowest level of the colon.

The sequence of events at this point gets murky. It is not clear whether tension achieved during ordinary motility events is sufficient in a closed chamber to pop diverticula through weak points in the musculature, or whether extraordinary stimuli or other additional factors resulting in weaknesses in the muscle coat are required. A stage of herniation of the mucosa into the thickened musculature, but not through it, is noted.

Once established, a diverticulum is remarkably stable over time. There can be progression in the numbers of diverticula and/or in the length of colon involved, but even this is not the rule (Parks, 1975). Observation of the appearance of diverticula at barium enema examination over periods of four to ten years (Hughes, 1969) has documented the basic stability of the diverticulum in terms of size, number, and distribution. The impression is one of diverticula formation as a result of a limited number of "events" rather than a continuous, steady, slow-moving process. This appearance is also consistent with a role for diverticula as a sort of safety valve to limit, but not normalize, the luminal pressures in a colonic segment. Parks and Connell (1969) and Smith and Shepherd (1976) demonstrated an increase in compliance in sigmoid colon muscle in segments involved with diverticular disease. This is in the face of every evidence of thickening and rigidity of the circular muscle with a gross loss of compliance. The original description by Howship (1824) of the morbid anatomy of the sigmoid musculature in diverticulosis is of muscle that is cartilaginous in consistency. It seems likely that the measured increase in compliance could be a result of the presence of the thin-walled, unsupported diverticular sac. Once sufficient diverticula form to provide an adequate capacity to vent the closed chamber and keep the pressure below a critical level, there is no stimulus for further growth of diverticula in size or number in that segment. A similar effect is achieved by longitudinal sigmoid myotomy, which has been used in treatment of sigmoid diverticular disease (Reilly, 1965).

Confirmation of this pathogenesis, if it is borne out, is of great clinical importance because of the implication that diverticular disease can be prevented as well as effectively managed to prevent the development of complications.

Diagnosis and Differential Diagnosis

Diagnosis of uncomplicated diverticulosis is always an incidental finding. Increasing use of fiberoptic sigmoidoscopy has led to direct diagnosis by observation of diverticulum openings, but such examinations are rarely capable of quantifying the extent of involvement with any degree of precision. The gold standard for diagnosis remains the barium enema x-ray, particularly when coupled with a late postevacuation film. Barium may be retained in diverticula for days. The most common reasons for ordering such studies are bleeding and nonspecific gastrointestinal tract symptoms. The finding of diverticula (even in association with apparent structural change) bears cautious interpretation. Symptoms of pain and disturbed bowel function, coupled with a barium-enema appearance of deformed bowel, have led to many unjustified diagnoses of diverticulitis when, in fact, the patient had diverticulosis with a shortened segment and thickening of the wall but no inflammation (Parks, et al., 1970). The symptoms were a result of attendant irritable bowel syndrome. The "-itis" diagnosis should be reserved for patients with evidence of active inflammation, such as fever, chills, leucocytosis, or a shift to the left in the differential white cell count. Even in the elderly patient with blunted responses to infection, inflammation will make itself manifest to the careful clinician.

Management of Uncomplicated Diverticulosis

Most of the literature concerning the management of uncomplicated diverticulosis seems concerned with the management of coincidental symptoms of irritable bowel syndrome. Fiber supplementation is the accepted mode of therapy. A number of controlled trials have been reported, and these are reviewed by Parks (1975). Generally, where fiber supplements have been adequate, results are excellent in terms of symptom control. None of these trials included in their design the evaluation of the effect of fiber supplementation on the prevention of the development of the complications of diverticulosis, bleeding, or peridiverticulitis. Without such evidence, the management of asymptomatic diverticulosis consists of benign neglect. This same lack of evidence leaves open the option to treat asymptomatic diverticulosis with fiber replacement. Complications, both bleeding and peridiverticulitis, are a result of inflammation—often minor inflammation—and are thought by some to be associated with inspissated intestinal contents within the diverticular sac. Reports of surgical treatment of diverticulosis with taeniomyotomy note spontaneous emptying of the diverticulum contents as the surgical division of the taenia progresses (Hodgson, 1973). This uncontrolled observation indirectly lends some credence to a preventive management program of asymptomatic disease.

Prevention of Diverticulosis

It is generally accepted that the basic underlying etiological factor in the development of diverticulosis is dietary fiber deficiency. This would imply that a significant change in fiber intake, either dietary fiber or supplementation, could alter the incidence of diverticulosis in the general population. Several factors make this relatively simple concept cumbersome to implement. While the evidence is scanty, the assumption is that dietary change or supplementation would need to be lifelong to effectively prevent the development of diverticula. Given the deeply rooted nature of traditional food preferences and the extensive commercial investment in food processing that removes fiber, the adoption of a significant dietary change by any major segment of the population seems unlikely. There are few data to suggest that fiber supplementation to prevent the development of diverticula would be cost effective, since the costs are associated with the development of complications. As a wellness concept, fiber supplementation has attracted a limited following.

COMPLICATIONS OF DIVERTICULAR DISEASE

Complications related to diverticula are generally a result of inflammation or bleeding. The inflammation may be limited to a single microperforation with peridiverticulitis, or it may be a life-threatening free perforation with peritonitis. Chronic inflammation with fistula or abscess may result, although the inflammation commonly resolves without sequelae. Bleeding may range from occult to exsanguinating hemorrhage.

Bleeding

As outlined above, diverticula have a constant and intimate relationship with the intestinal wall vasculature. The penetrating diverticulum lifts the nutrient artery (Figs. 6–2 and 6–3) and its attendant vein. This close relationship with an arterial vessel produces an opportunity for substantial bleeding. The frequency with which diverticular bleeding occurs is an enigma despite intense interest and a number of studies. Clearly much of the attention is focused on gross bleeding. Its diagnosis is simple and dramatic, although its differential diagnosis may be difficult. Occult bleeding lacks the drama of presentation but has potential clinical significance. Epidemiological studies that are both unbiased in terms of selection and invasive enough to be accurate are not at hand. Thus, the relative significance of diverticular bleeding remains a question.

A second complicating feature has been the emerging understanding of the range of etiologies for gross rectal bleeding. Many of the earlier studies (Noer, et al., 1962; Behringer & Albright, 1973) preceded the studies that demonstrated the role of vascular ectasias as bleeding lesions in the colon, particularly in the elderly (Boley, et al., 1979; 1977a). It now seems clear that these interesting, acquired lesions are common sources for rectal bleeding in the elderly, and some changes in diagnosis and management are implied.

Pathology and Pathologic Physiology

When a bleeding diverticulum is the diagnosis and the presentation has been that of gross bleeding, then the source is usually arterial rupture in a single diverticulum in the right colon (Meyers, et al., 1976). Arterial bleeding from a diverticulum in the colon is usually through a blowout located in the dome of the diverticulum and does not seem to be directly related to an active inflammatory process (Meyers, et al., 1973; 1976). Nonarterial bleeding does occur and seems most frequently associated with mucosal inflammation—diverticulitis or colitis—involving the highly vascular ring of mucosa that develops surrounding the opening of the diverticulum (Meyers, et al., 1973).

Meyers and colleagues (1976) have done a careful and comprehensive evaluation of ten patients with bleeding diverticulosis. They report that the involved vasa rectae in the bleeding diverticulum characteristically demonstrate intimal thickening, alteration, and usually duplication of the internal elastic lamella and attenuation of the media. These changes involve only the arterial wall adjacent to the diverticular lumen. The change is eccentric and segmental. Changes are limited to the bleeding diverticulum. Vasa rectae in adjacent but nonbleeding diverticula show little intimal thickening or other change. The development of intimal thickening in an arterial wall is often a nonspecific, observed response of the arterial wall to a variety of injuries. Unfortunately at this point, data are replaced by speculation, and the nature of the injury is unknown. The eccentric and segmental location in the arterial wall would indicate that the injury is related to the specific diverticulum rather than to the process of diverticular formation, since only one of many diverticula is usually affected. Trauma or inflammation associated with concretions of intestinal content within the diverticulum is often implicated, but the colonic contents on the right side of the colon are fluid and are far less likely to form concretions than on the left side. Right-sided diverticula are wider in the neck and are thus less likely to plug. Histological evidence of inflammation is lacking, and thus ulceration of the mucosa followed by erosion of an underlying artery is an unlikely sequence as a cause for bleeding. Mechanical factors and/or toxins have been postulated, but there is little evidence either for or against this implication. The lack of a definable mechanism makes long-term preventive therapy with fiber supplements after diverticula have formed speculative at best.

Clinical Presentation

Gross rectal bleeding from arterial rupture within a diverticulum usually has a dramatic and abrupt presentation. Often the patient is without any symptoms referable to the digestive tract prior to the passage of a grossly bloody stool. The bleeding is from a very small artery and is steady but not so brisk that it invariably results in shock. Even though the vasoreactivity of elderly patients is often characterized as sluggish—an explanation for the increased frequency of postural hypotension and postural vertigo—given time, it is effective. Slow bleeding into a capacious colon may be surprisingly symptom-free until the production of a large bloody stool. When symptoms do occur, they are as likely to be those of hypovolemia as those of abdominal distress. Abdominal complaints that do occur are usually confined to lower abdominal cramping antecedent to the evacuation of a bloody stool.

Spontaneous remission of the bleeding is the rule (Quinn, 1961). Bleeding will usually continue for as long as two days. Whether this represents a continuous ooze or intermittent bleeding may be critical in the selection of diagnostic studies but is often beyond the range of clinical sensitivity. Once bleeding stops, approximately one quarter of the patients may anticipate an early or delayed rebleed (McGuire &

Haynes, 1972). The likelihood of another rebleed increases dramatically with each succeeding episode (Gennaro & Rosemond, 1973).

Diagnosis and Differential Diagnosis

Definitive diagnosis depends upon the demonstration of the bleeding site. Angiography (much less commonly surgery or colonoscopy) can do this. Often the clinical circumstances permit only a presumptive diagnosis. Several of the diagnostic maneuvers are limited in their scope to a specific clinical setting. An orderly approach to the diagnostic process is essential since the most powerful—angiography and colonoscopy—are invasive and are of limited tolerance in the frail elderly. An algorithm outlining one approach to evaluation of gross rectal bleeding is presented in Figure 6–4.

The first concern is for the stability of the patient, and with bleeding

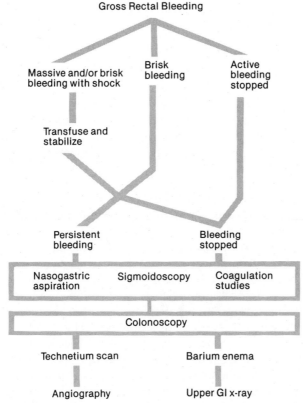

Figure 6–4. Algorithm outlining an approach to the evaluation of gross rectal bleeding.

the cardiovascular status is the focus. The margin of clinical reserve is often compromised in the elderly, with diminished cardiac reserve, decreased renal function, arteriosclerotic changes in the peripheral vessels, and confusion. Care must be individualized.

Diagnostic maneuvers are often incorporated with the assessment of clinical status. Nasogastric aspiration will give a quick but incomplete reading on the presence of upper gastrointestinal hemorrhage, either peptic or variceal. Digital rectal examination, anoscopy, and/or procto-sigmoidoscopy can turn up chronic ulcerative colitis, Crohn's disease of the colon, low-lying carcinoma, and massively bleeding hemorrhoids. With a simple enema preparation and use of the flexible instrument, the examination is surprisingly well tolerated even in the frail elderly. In addition to the blood count and panel chemistries, it is important to obtain laboratory evaluation of clotting factors. Clotting abnormalities may be a primary cause of the rectal bleeding or may just add to the management difficulty of bleeding from other sources.

If bleeding appears to continue and the patient's condition permits, an attempt should be made to visualize the bleeding site. Where available, the use of ^{99}Tc-labeled autologous red blood cells may confirm the continued presence of active bleeding in questionable cases and may guide the focus of angiographic studies if they are undertaken (Winzelberg, et al., 1981).

Selective angiography can identify the site of the bleeding divertic-ulum if bleeding remains brisk enough to permit accumulation of visible contrast in the diverticulum and/or the lumen of the colon. While diverticular bleeding is most common from the right side of the colon, bleeding diverticula in other colonic segments are not excluded. Selec-tive studies of celiac, superior, and inferior mesenteric arteries may be necessary to find the bleeder or to complete the study. Even though such studies may be quickly performed and have a low rate of compli-cation, they may stretch the tolerance of the elderly patient. In the event that a bleeding site is identified, then the selective arteriography catheter does offer an avenue for therapeutic intervention either by infusion of vasoconstrictor or by selective embolization.

When active bleeding does not persist or angiography fails to identify a bleeding site, colonoscopy is the next procedure in order of precedence. The critical limiting feature for colonoscopy is the success with which one can clean and prepare the colon for inspection. Even in the elderly patient, lavage with a nonabsorbable solution has a high rate of success and a good margin of safety. The diagnostic accuracy exceeds 90 per cent (Gostout, 1988). Endoscopic identification of a site of hemorrhage whether from a diverticulum or from a vascular ectasia may not only resolve a diagnostic dilemma but also afford an opportunity for therapeutic intervention with one of the various modalities for coagulation of a vascular lesion.

Barium contrast x-rays rank lowest in the order of diagnostic maneuvers simply because, while they can tell you where there is a lesion that could bleed, they cannot tell you if it is bleeding. Once barium has been introduced into the digestive tract, angiographic studies are effectively precluded for intervals that may last up to one week. Barium in the colon adds to the difficulty of cleansing the colon for endoscopic studies.

Gross rectal bleeding can result from upper gastrointestinal hemorrhage, either peptic or variceal. Both are relatively uncommon presentations of a common problem of the elderly. Digestive tract neoplasms that can bleed, particularly carcinoma of the colon, increase in frequency of presentation in the elderly. Idiopathic inflammatory bowel disease, including chronic ulcerative colitis, ulcerative proctitis, and Crohn's disease, all can have an initial presentation late in life. Acquired vascular malformations (vascular ectasias, angiodysplasia, arteriovenous malformations) share with diverticula a leading role in the etiology of rectal bleeding in the elderly. Management options vary with the differing etiologies for rectal bleeding. Diagnostic maneuvers often offer opportunities for management intervention. Most of these procedures are in the hands of subspecialists. To optimize care, the responsible attending physician has a demanding responsibility in the selection of the sequence of diagnostic maneuvers.

Management

As discussed above, bleeding episodes in most patients will stop spontaneously. These patients require only the appropriate medical intervention with supportive measures. Restoration of vascular volume with either intravenous fluids or transfusion must be tempered by the compromised cardiac reserve that often occurs in the elderly. The traditional clear liquid diet seems more a hedge against the potential for rebleed and the need for further work-up than a therapy of any real benefit. Early ambulation, while desirable, must always be governed by the patient's cardiac reserve.

When active bleeding continues and the source is identified by angiography, there is the opportunity to utilize selective intraarterial vasopressin to control the hemorrhage. Reported results are excellent in terms of control of acute bleeding. Athanasoulis and coworkers (1975) reported control of hemorrhage in 22 of 24 well-studied patients. Twelve of these patients received no further therapy, and three of this group of twelve rebled after some months. Each of the episodes of rebleeding requires individual assessment in terms of the frequency with which it occurs, the intervals between bleeding episodes, the patient's past experience with vasopressin, and the current full spectrum of other medical problems. The excellent response to vasopressin is attributed to the nature of the bleed, which, as outlined above, is usually from a single small artery rather than from diffuse or multiple bleeders.

Reported side effects of vasopressin include serious cardiovascular compromise with angina, EKG changes of ischemia, myocardial infarction, vascular collapse, and arrhythmias. High doses of vasopressin and/or bolus injection are more likely to produce these serious untoward reactions than the slow infusion used for diverticular hemorrhage.

If vasopressin fails to control the hemorrhage, then management usually requires surgical intervention. Transcatheter embolization to control massive hemorrhage has been reported (Goldberger & Bookstein, 1977), but its use is not widespread. When the bleeding site has been identified by angiography, then segmental colectomy will suffice. When a bleeding site cannot be specifically identified and the bleeding is severe and/or intermittent, then surgical intervention with hemicolectomy or subtotal colectomy may be required. This is usually a last ditch effort to control hemorrhage.

Diverticulitis

Inflammation associated with diverticula is the most common complication of diverticulosis. Acute and chronic forms occur, and diverticulitis can lead to several secondary complications, e.g., fistula, peritonitis, or obstruction.

Pathology and Pathologic Physiology

Most of the inflammatory disease related to diverticula occurs on the left side in the sigmoid and descending colon. The open-mouthed right-sided diverticula and the semifluid contents of the right colon interact to produce eccentric damage to the small arteries and bleeding associated with the diverticula in proximal colon, whereas the narrower necked diverticula in the distal colon exposed to the semisolid contents respond by becoming inflamed. In contrast studies diverticula are seen to fill and empty themselves with barium. Emptying is often delayed and forms the basis for diagnosis by delayed postevacuation films after barium enema. Surgeons often observe feces-filled diverticula, and, as noted above, these will empty spontaneously as taeniomyotomy progresses (Hodgson, 1973). Retained inspissated fecal material is a factor in the development of inflammation (Thompson & Patel, 1986). This leads to the speculation that while abnormal pressure relationships induced by a fiber-deficient diet lead to the formation of diverticula, it is slow transit with dehydration of feces which forms hard scybala within the diverticula that sets the stage for inflammatory complications. Diverticulitis with free perforation has been reported in defunctionalized colon distal to a colostomy (Dardik, et al., 1964). In this case inspissated mucoliths were implicated as a cause. In the intact bowel, if dehydration of the fecal mass is the cause, then fiber supplementation may have a salutary effect in preventing inflammation by increasing the fecal water and keeping the stool soft.

Whatever the mechanism, the inflammation begins as a microperforation usually at the tip of the diverticulum. This stage of microabscess is often referred to in the European literature as phlegmonous diverticulitis (Hughes, 1975). This can enlarge to involve adjacent colonic tissues and produce an abscess, can perforate into the peritoneum and cause peritonitis, or can dissect to result in abscess and/or fistula formation. Usually the process remains localized and resolves with medical management, but it does leave behind a residual scar. With recurrent attacks (and recurrence, while not the rule, is not uncommon), scarring may produce deformity in the bowel and can result in either partial or complete intestinal obstruction. The accumulation of scar tissue facilitates the walling off of abscesses, a characteristic of late complications. Aggressive inflammatory responses during initial attacks may be more likely to end in free perforation with a critically ill, toxic patient. Inflamed colon may become adherent to adjacent viscera, and perforation of an abscess may lead to a fistula. Vesicocolonic fistulas seem most common. Perforation back into the intestine may result in a clinically silent fistula, unless a large excluded loop is formed with resultant malabsorption. The abscess may dissect through the pericolic tissues to form a fistula. Less commonly fistula may dissect to the skin or the vagina.

Clinical Presentation

The three hallmarks of the clinical presentation of acute diverticulitis are abdominal pain, fever, and leucocytosis with an increased percentage of polymorphonuclear cells. The pain is crampy and localized in the left lower quadrant, reflecting the usual sigmoid location of the diverticulitis. The pain is highly variable in its severity. The sigmoid has some mobility, and the localization of the pain and its referral pattern will show much variability. Inflamed diverticula adjacent to small intestine or urinary bladder can change the presentation deceptively. In its milder presentation, the pain has little to distinguish itself from that in irritable bowel syndrome or ischemia. Should the inflammation lie adjacent to the bladder, the patient may complain of urgency or frequency. Usually there is an associated change in bowel habit, often constipation and irregularity but occasionally diarrhea. Additional gastrointestinal signs and symptoms include anorexia, nausea, vomiting, and abdominal distention. Distention can be due to ileus or intestinal obstruction.

Physical examination will often reveal focal abdominal tenderness with or without evidence of peritoneal irritation. Often a mass, or at least a sense of fullness, may be palpated in the left lower quadrant. Occasionally pain will be demonstrated only during pelvic or rectal exam. Unfortunately, pain, tenderness, and even a palpable mass are not uncommon accompaniments of irritable bowel syndrome, and more objective evidence of inflammation needs to be sought. Fever is not a feature of irritable bowel syndrome. Elevations may be mild or hectic, and chills and sweats can be experienced. The well-known propensity of the elderly to mount only a muted febrile response to significant infection adds the requirement for careful procedure in taking temperatures—regular recalibration of the electronic thermometers and frequent readings to document elevations in these patients.

Leucocytosis and/or a shift to the left in the differential count are also objective signs of inflammation, but these signs tend to have a sluggish response in some elderly patients. The presence of red and white cells in the urinary sediment, particularly in the absence of significant bacilluria, may be an indicator of inflammation in a loop of sigmoid adjacent to the bladder.

Perhaps the most striking feature is the high degree of variability in the pattern of presentation from patient to patient. A full blown attack of diverticulitis is a straightforward diagnosis, but differentiation of mild attacks, particularly from irritable bowel syndrome, can be a challenging task. The same problem looms with patients who have acute exacerbation of chronic diverticulitis. Often mild lower abdominal symptoms persist between acute attacks. It is never clear whether the cramping discomfort, tenderness, and irregularity reflect the fibrosis and scarring of repeated bouts of inflammation, the incidental occurrence of irritable bowel syndrome, or some residual smoldering low grade inflammation. The occurrence of fever, even low grade elevations, and leucocytosis may be the only reliable guides to therapeutic intervention.

Diagnosis and Differential Diagnosis

As outlined above, the diagnosis rests with identification of objective signs of active inflammation. In addition to the physical and laboratory findings already mentioned, there are several other helpful procedures. Flat and upright x-rays can give evidence of ileus. They also permit a look for free air under the diaphragm. Gentle sigmoidoscopy with the fiberoptic instrument, avoiding air insufflation, can rule out the diagnosis of colitis or low-lying tumor. These exams, while revealing, are often incomplete and bear repeating after convalescence. Sigmoidoscopy should not be a routine procedure during acute attacks. It should be reserved for those cases in which the diagnosis remains unclear and there is need for urgent choice between alternative therapies. Colonoscopy can usually be deferred until acute symptoms have subsided.

The use of barium enema x-ray examination for diagnosis of potential acute diverticulitis has been a focus of some controversy. Concern that barium instillation is likely to lead to perforation seems largely unfounded (Nicholas, et al., 1972). The procedure is safe in skilled, careful hands, but the diagnostic benefit is somewhat more limited than was earlier believed. Extravasation of barium outside of the lumen into an abscess cavity or down a fistulous tract is helpful in the evaluation of extent and activity of disease and in the confirmation of diverticula. Barium enema has not proved helpful in the differentiation of diverticulitis from diverticulosis. One British study (Parks, et al., 1970) found substantial lack of correlation between independent readings of several radiologists and significant variance between the radiological diagnoses and the findings when examined by a pathologist. The conclusion was that barium enema is simply not an accurate indicator of the presence of inflammation-complicating diverticular disease. Even though the risk of barium enema during acute diverticulitis is small, there does not seem to be sufficient diagnostic benefit to warrant its use.

The availability of computerized axial tomography (CAT scan) as a noninvasive tool for accurate localization of abscesses effectively removes barium enema from the diagnostic armamentarium for acute diverticulitis. It does retain an important role in the evaluation of the status of the colon and in the search for fistula once the acute attack has subsided.

The differential diagnosis includes inflammatory bowel disease, carcinoma of the colon, ischemic colitis, and occasionally rectal abscess. All are readily excluded by selection of the appropriate procedure as long as one remembers to consider these possibilities in the first place. The much more difficult differential between diverticulosis and diverticulitis has been discussed above.

Management

The spectrum of disease ranges from mild abdominal cramping with a low grade fever to patients who are toxic, febrile, and incapacitated with pain. A mild attack (that is, pain not requiring prescription analgesia, no evidence of ileus or obstruction, and only a low grade fever) can usually be managed outside of the hospital with appropriate antibiotics, clear liquids, and rest. Patients who require analgesia or give evidence of functional or focal obstruction are best admitted to the hospital. Persistent nausea and vomiting, hectic fevers, and signs of toxicity are also indicators for hospital admission.

In-hospital management usually implies a need for intravenous fluids and bowel rest. Antibiotic therapy is always in order for the hospitalized patient. Since one is dealing with a mixed flora from the bowel, the initial selection of an antibiotic is empirical. Ampicillin or one of the cephalosporins is usually the first choice. Blood cultures taken before the antibiotics are started may permit later fine tuning of the antibiotic regimen. A failure to respond should prompt a search for a secondary complication, such as abscess or perforation, as well as possible revision of the antibiotic selection.

Diverticulitis is an infectious complication, and there are both diagnostic and therapeutic concerns particular to the aged. Other coincident medical problems may so narrow the patient's reserve that even mild diverticulitis warrants admission. This is particularly true when dehydration or electrolyte imbalance occurs in patients being treated for cardiac failure or arrhythmia. The physiological response to infection in the elderly may be sluggish or attenuated. Once the diagnosis has been entertained, therapy should be early and vigorous even though physical findings seem minimal.

Surgical intervention during an attack of acute diverticulitis is called for in the face of perforation with peritonitis, obstruction, and failure of resolution of an abscess after initiation of adequate antibiotic chemotherapy. The risks of surgery are high in the case of any patient with an acute attack, and particularly so in elderly patients, hence its limitation to essentially life-threatening settings. In most cases the surgery represents the beginning of a two- or three-stage procedure. The initial surgical intervention is limited to the least procedure that can stabilize the patient. Usually this is a defunctionalizing colostomy combined with peritoneal lavage, resection of the perforated colon, internal drainage of the abscess if feasible, or just the colostomy alone for obstruction. Once the infection has been brought under control, surgery to perform definitive procedures can also be carried out in stages if necessary.

The clear indications for elective surgery are the management of fistula and the correction of partial obstruction. Recurrent attacks that are frequent and disabling and that do not respond to medical management are also candidates for resection. However, this is always subject to some controversy, since the endpoint is subjective. Careful follow-up surveys (Bolt & Hughes 1966; Parks & Connell, 1970) indicate that one quarter or more of the patients resected because of symptoms will continue to have lower abdominal sympton. surgery. The diagnosis of recurrent attacks of diverticulitis sho. made on the strength of objective evidence of inflammation.

Medical management of chronic recurrent attacks is essenti. limited to the attempt to prevent their occurrence by provision of high fiber diet. Fiber supplementation, usually in the form of bran, should not be begun until acute inflammation has subsided. The rational use of bran and other fiber supplements has been discussed in Chapter 5. Bran not only provides bulk, which seems to lower the intraluminal pressures, but also increases fecal water to keep the stool soft. Reduced intraluminal pressures permit easier evacuation of the diverticular sacs, reduced muscle tension in the wall leaves the neck of the diverticulum open to facilitate emptying, and the increase in fecal water prevents inspissation of fecaliths within the diverticular sac. One study on the effect of high fiber diets in complications of diverticula has been published (Hyland & Taylor, 1980), with the conclusion that high fiber diets do protect against recurrent complications. The results were impressive, but the study lacked controls. Confirmation by a controlled study is awaited.

Surgical management of chronic recurrent attacks may involve resection, as discussed above, or the use of myotomy. Both longitudinal sigmoid myotomy and transverse taeniomyotomy have been employed. In skilled surgical hands and with careful selection of patients, both surgical techniques show good success (Hodgson, 1973; Reilly, 1975). Neither procedure is widely available.

Much of the above may seem like an indictment against surgical management of chronic recurrent diverticulitis, and this is not intended. The success of newer approaches to medical management has narrowed the number of surgical candidates. With careful matching of patient and procedure, many who have not benefited from medical therapy can be helped. It does the patient with chronic recurrent diverticulitis no service to persist in ineffectual medical management, while scarring progresses, in a misplaced attempt to avoid surgery. When surgical intervention finally comes, it has greater hazard and may offer less complete amelioration because of the delay.

Secondary Complications

Secondary complications include fistula, obstruction, and abscess. All of them represent extensions in scale of the primary infectious process.

Abscess

The initial lesion in acute diverticulitis is a microabscess that usually forms at the tip of the diverticulum. If this abscess enlarges beyond the muscular wall of the colon into the mesocolic fat, it becomes a pericolic abscess (Hughes, 1975). The abscess wall may incorporate any adjacent structure, small or large intestine, bladder, uterus, omentum, or parietal peritoneum. Resolution of the abscess is possible with appropriate antibiotic chemotherapy; however, the larger the abscess, the more likely it is to require drainage for complete resolution.

Drainage is usually spontaneous and back into the bowel lumen. The original inflammatory tract is often the line of least resistance. Pus may dissect along the bowel before returning to the lumen. If the original inflammatory tract from lumen to abscess remains, usually termed a communicating abscess, then an enteric fistula will form. More distant loops of intestine, particularly the mobile small intestine, may become incorporated into the abscess wall. Drainage can then occur into the ileum or jejunum, and if the original tract from colon to abscess remains intact, an ileocolic or jejunocolic fistula can result. Abscess may discharge into adjacent organs, such as the bladder, or through the abdominal wall. With each location there is the risk of fistula formation.

Evacuation into the peritoneal cavity will result in peritonitis. If the original tract from the colon to the abscess has sealed, then this noncommunicating peritonitis is readily managed with antibiotics and drainage (Hughes, 1975). A communicating peritonitis with ongoing fecal soilage usually requires more vigorous surgical management, with some procedure to resolve the perforation as well as to defunctionalize the distal colon.

Adequate drainage without fistula formation usually permits complete resolution of the abscess. In years gone by, abscess was a difficult diagnosis. It was simply one of several possible space-occupying lesions located in an area diagnostically difficult to approach. With the advent of the CAT scan and ultrasonography, there are now noninvasive and highly accurate tools to use in the identification of abscess. These modalities make it possible to follow the resolution of a collection and the identification of failures to respond. Failure of resolution of an abscess with appropriate antibiotic therapy, particularly in the face of clinical evidence of advancing toxicity, merits the consideration of immediate surgical intervention to effect drainage or resect the abscess.

Fistula

Fistula may form as a result of spontaneous or surgical drainage of a communicating abscess. Generally this is in a clinical setting and is an exacerbation of the diverticulitis with pain and fever. The fistula may also be the presenting event without the antecedent signs and symptoms of acute diverticulitis. This seems to be a matter of timing

rather than of some intr...
kind of fistula.

The most common clinica... ...e in the pathog...
diverticulitis is often silent; the p... ...(Henderson & Small, 1969), and m...fistulae are vesicoc... mechanism is related to the relatively...s that of recurrent c... sigmoid colon. When this short segme...ost often affected. 1... involved with diverticulitis, it is so position...gment of the pelvic to the posterior wall of the bladder. A sm... ...sigmoid becomes evacuating through the wall of the bladder will c...necting abscess become adherent substantial prior experience with diverticulitis in th...e fistula. Any shorten the colon and prevent contact with the bladde...ent would of a past history of symptomatic inflammation is esse... The lack pathophysiology of the development of this fistula. Male pre...m...nce to the is explained by the protective cover which the uterus offers to t...e b...k of the bladder in females.

The clinical presentation is that of recurrent cystitis with dysuria and frequency of urination. Pneumaturia is a frequent finding in men but is rarely described in women. This is due to the fact that pneumaturia is observed but not felt. In the upright patient, the gas bubble in the bladder sits atop the urine and its passage follows the passage of urine (Henderson & Small, 1969). The urethra is no more perceptive than the anal canal (see Chapter 5), and liquid and gas "feel" the same to the mucosa. Males generally observe their urinary stream while females do not, and thus only men are aware that they are passing "air." Fortunately, as was mentioned, women have some protection from fistula in the first place.

Diagnosis can be difficult. Generally the pressures within the colon are higher than the intravesical pressure (Small & Smith, 1975). For this reason the presentation is usually that of a urinary tract abnormality. In the elderly male with a tendency for outlet obstruction as benign prostatic hypertrophy develops, passage of urine through the rectum can occur. Fistula is in the differential diagnosis of watery diarrhea.

Cystoscopy may show a patch of cystitis on the bladder wall, but only rarely will it visualize the opening of the fistulous tract. Cystograms with radiopaque media rarely visualize the tract. An approach from the bowel is similarly unrewarding. Barium does not regularly visualize the tract, and the tract opening is also not distinctive on sigmoidoscopy. An upright x-ray may show the air in the bladder, particularly if done immediately after a sigmoidoscopy. A high index of suspicion and pneumaturia are the two best clues to the diagnosis. Surgical resection is the only practical approach to management.

Fistula may form to the small intestine, either ileum or jejunum. Ileocolic fistula involving distal ileum are often completely silent and

...ma examination. As the entry of
are incidental findings at ...alabsorption may become evident.
the fistulous tract creep...can eventually lead to megaloblastic
Bypass of the recept...rs for bile acid resorption can spill bile
anemia. Bypass of t...when deconjugated by bacteria, results in
acids into the colo...management will suffice with appropriate
diarrhea. Often ...d binding resins for bile acids. Should these
replacement the...option for surgical resection. Diagnosis may be
fail, then ther...rly with ileocolic fistula where differentiation from
confusing, p...s a concern.
Crohn's dis...ous and colovaginal fistula are uncommon. With a
Colo...fistula, one is always concerned about carcinoma of the
colovagi...an etiology. Crohn's disease is also a consideration. Postirra-
cervix...itis with fistula should be apparent from history.
dia...n c...

Obstruction

Intestinal obstruction during an acute attack of diverticulitis may
be due to adynamic ileus or to obstruction by an inflammatory mass
(Hughes, 1975). In chronic disease, scarring and kinking of the lumen
may produce partial or complete obstruction. The partial obstruction in
this case may fluctuate as the inflammatory process waxes and wanes.
Either kind of obstruction can involve the small or the large intestine.
Complete obstruction is an emergency readily recognized in a patient
with distention, vomiting, and air fluid levels in the bowel on upright
x-ray of the abdomen. Peritoneal soiling with resultant adynamic ileus
must be differentiated from obstruction by an inflammatory mass.

Obstruction without peritonitis should be managed conservatively,
with the patient placed NPO to give bowel rest parenteral fluids
administered to maintain hydration and electrolyte balance. The patient
needs to be followed in a serial fashion, with the anticipation that the
control of the inflammation will permit relief of the obstruction. Urgent
surgery, particularly in the elderly, is always at the price of increased
morbidity and mortality. Once the obstruction is relieved and the
patient is stabilized, definitive evaluation for the possibility of surgical
intervention is in order. The management of obstruction secondary to
ileus associated with peritonitis has been discussed above.

RIGHT-SIDED DIVERTICULOSIS

Most of the discussion above concerning the pathologic physiology
of the development of diverticula is based on change observed grossly
and microscopically in the sigmoid and distal descending colon. Diverticula do occur on the right side of the colon and except for the final

common path, which must be an increased intraluminal pressure within a closed chamber of the colon which exceeds the critical level at which weak points in the colonic circular muscle fail and a mucosal diverticulum is formed, the underlying mechanism is probably different. Generally right-sided diverticula are found in conjunction with extensive left-sided disease (Morson, 1975). Thickening of the muscle, not as marked as it is on the left, and accentuation of the haustra, again not as marked as on the left but enough to produce hypersegmentation in a gross specimen, has been reported by Morson (1975). Studies of elastosis have been confined to material from the left colon.

An additional form of diverticular disease, involving the right side of the colon without sigmoid involvement, has been described and seems to represent another separate entity. This is the predominant form of diverticular disease among Orientals in the Pacific basin (Peck, et al., 1968). The underlying cause of these diverticula is a mystery. The gross specimens are reported (Perry & Morson, 1971) to show only equivocal changes in the muscle and slight accentuation of the haustra. There was lymphoid hyperplasia surrounding the orifices of the diverticula but no indication whether this was cause or effect. This also seems to be a problem of the elderly. The clinical presentation can be either acute diverticulitis or bleeding.

A third form of right-sided diverticulosis is solitary cecal diverticulum. These often appear to be congenital diverticula, although acquired diverticulum also occurs. Inflammation and bleeding can occur. This lesion tends to present in a younger age group.

SIMPLE MASSED DIVERTICULOSIS

Diverticula are found in many patients without any evidence of muscular thickening, haustral accentuation, or shortening of the colon. Most often these are incidental findings at the time of a barium enema, but on occasion these diverticula can bleed or become inflamed. Scattered single diverticula are common. Occasionally the colon will be lined with diverticula over a segment or over the entire colon (Fig. 6–5). While the appearance is arresting, these are not often a symptomatic clinical problem. The underlying mechanism for their formation is obscure; they are a phenomenon of the aging process. The speculation is that these are formed at unusual weak points in the bowel wall where the critical pressure for the herniation of mucosa is close to pressures ordinarily found in the colon.

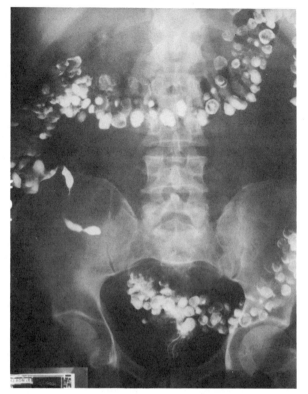

Figure 6–5. Radiograph showing simple massed diverticulosis. The retained barium in the diverticula remains from a barium study performed two weeks previously. (Courtesy of Dr. Peter Meyers).

GIANT SIGMOID DIVERTICULUM (AIR CYST, GIANT COLONIC DIVERTICULUM)

Giant sigmoid diverticulum is thought to be a complication of sigmoid diverticulosis, but because of its unusual presentation and its unknown pathogenesis, it will be treated separately. It has a predilection for the aged, which is no more than a reflection of its constant association with sigmoid diverticulosis. It is not often seen. While the usual name for the lesion is giant sigmoid diverticulum, it is occasionally described in other locations in the colon, notably the transverse colon.

Pathology and Pathologic Physiology

A giant diverticulum is defined as a large (5 to 30 cm in diameter) cystic structure usually arising from the sigmoid colon (Moss, 1975). Connection with the lumen of the colon may or may not remain doscopy with the fiberoptic instrument, avoiding air insufflation, can rule out the diagnosis of colitis or low-lying tumor. These exams, while revealing, are often incomplete and bear repeating after convalescence. Sigmoidoscopy should not be a routine procedure during acute attacks. It should be reserved for those cases in which the diagnosis remains unclear and there is need for urgent choice between alternative therapies. Colonoscopy can usually be deferred until acute symptoms have subsided.

The use of barium enema x-ray examination for diagnosis of potential acute diverticulitis has been a focus of some controversy. Concern that barium instillation is likely to lead to perforation seems largely unfounded (Nicholas, et al., 1972). The procedure is safe in skilled, careful hands, but the diagnostic benefit is somewhat more limited than was earlier believed. Extravasation of barium outside of the lumen into an abscess cavity or down a fistulous tract is helpful in the evaluation of extent and activity of disease and in the confirmation of diverticula. Barium enema has not proved helpful in the differentiation of diverticulitis from diverticulosis. One British study (Parks, et al., 1970) found substantial lack of correlation between independent readings of several radiologists and significant variance between the radiological diagnoses and the findings when examined by a pathologist. The conclusion was that barium enema is simply not an accurate indicator of the presence of inflammation-complicating diverticular disease. Even though the risk of barium enema during acute diverticulitis is small, there does not seem to be sufficient diagnostic benefit to warrant its use.

The availability of computerized axial tomography (CAT scan) as a noninvasive tool for accurate localization of abscesses effectively removes barium enema from the diagnostic armamentarium for acute diverticulitis. It does retain an important role in the evaluation of the status of the colon and in the search for fistula once the acute attack has subsided.

The differential diagnosis includes inflammatory bowel disease, carcinoma of the colon, ischemic colitis, and occasionally rectal abscess. All are readily excluded by selection of the appropriate procedure as long as one remembers to consider these possibilities in the first place. The much more difficult differential between diverticulosis and diverticulitis has been discussed above.

Management

The spectrum of disease ranges from mild abdominal cramping with a low grade fever to patients who are toxic, febrile, and incapacitated with pain. A mild attack (that is, pain not requiring prescription analgesia, no evidence of ileus or obstruction, and only a low grade fever) can usually be managed outside of the hospital with appropriate antibiotics, clear liquids, and rest. Patients who require analgesia or give evidence of functional or focal obstruction are best admitted to the hospital. Persistent nausea and vomiting, hectic fevers, and signs of toxicity are also indicators for hospital admission.

In-hospital management usually implies a need for intravenous fluids and bowel rest. Antibiotic therapy is always in order for the hospitalized patient. Since one is dealing with a mixed flora from the bowel, the initial selection of an antibiotic is empirical. Ampicillin or one of the cephalosporins is usually the first choice. Blood cultures taken before the antibiotics are started may permit later fine tuning of the antibiotic regimen. A failure to respond should prompt a search for a secondary complication, such as abscess or perforation, as well as possible revision of the antibiotic selection.

Diverticulitis is an infectious complication, and there are both diagnostic and therapeutic concerns particular to the aged. Other coincident medical problems may so narrow the patient's reserve that even mild diverticulitis warrants admission. This is particularly true when dehydration or electrolyte imbalance occurs in patients being treated for cardiac failure or arrhythmia. The physiological response to infection in the elderly may be sluggish or attenuated. Once the diagnosis has been entertained, therapy should be early and vigorous even though physical findings seem minimal.

Surgical intervention during an attack of acute diverticulitis is called for in the face of perforation with peritonitis, obstruction, and failure of resolution of an abscess after initiation of adequate antibiotic chemotherapy. The risks of surgery are high in the case of any patient with an acute attack, and particularly so in elderly patients, hence its limitation to essentially life-threatening settings. In most cases the surgery represents the beginning of a two- or three-stage procedure. The initial surgical intervention is limited to the least procedure that can stabilize the patient. Usually this is a defunctionalizing colostomy combined with peritoneal lavage, resection of the perforated colon, internal drainage of the abscess if feasible, or just the colostomy alone for obstruction. Once the infection has been brought under control, surgery to perform definitive procedures can also be carried out in stages if necessary.

The clear indications for elective surgery are the management of fistula and the correction of partial obstruction. Recurrent attacks that are frequent and disabling and that do not respond to medical management are also candidates for resection. However, this is always subject to some controversy, since the endpoint is subjective. Careful follow-up surveys (Bolt & Hughes 1966; Parks & Connell, 1970) indicate that one quarter or more of the patients resected because of symptoms will continue to have lower abdominal sympton surgery. The diagnosis of recurrent attacks of diverticulitis sho made on the strength of objective evidence of inflammation.

Medical management of chronic recurrent attacks is essenti limited to the attempt to prevent their occurrence by provision of high fiber diet. Fiber supplementation, usually in the form of bran, should not be begun until acute inflammation has subsided. The rational use of bran and other fiber supplements has been discussed in Chapter 5. Bran not only provides bulk, which seems to lower the intraluminal pressures, but also increases fecal water to keep the stool soft. Reduced intraluminal pressures permit easier evacuation of the diverticular sacs, reduced muscle tension in the wall leaves the neck of the diverticulum open to facilitate emptying, and the increase in fecal water prevents inspissation of fecaliths within the diverticular sac. One study on the effect of high fiber diets in complications of diverticula has been published (Hyland & Taylor, 1980), with the conclusion that high fiber diets do protect against recurrent complications. The results were impressive, but the study lacked controls. Confirmation by a controlled study is awaited.

Surgical management of chronic recurrent attacks may involve resection, as discussed above, or the use of myotomy. Both longitudinal sigmoid myotomy and transverse taeniomyotomy have been employed. In skilled surgical hands and with careful selection of patients, both surgical techniques show good success (Hodgson, 1973; Reilly, 1975). Neither procedure is widely available.

Much of the above may seem like an indictment against surgical management of chronic recurrent diverticulitis, and this is not intended. The success of newer approaches to medical management has narrowed the number of surgical candidates. With careful matching of patient and procedure, many who have not benefited from medical therapy can be helped. It does the patient with chronic recurrent diverticulitis no service to persist in ineffectual medical management, while scarring progresses, in a misplaced attempt to avoid surgery. When surgical intervention finally comes, it has greater hazard and may offer less complete amelioration because of the delay.

Secondary Complications

Secondary complications include fistula, obstruction, and abscess. All of them represent extensions in scale of the primary infectious process.

Abscess

The initial lesion in acute diverticulitis is a microabscess that usually forms at the tip of the diverticulum. If this abscess enlarges beyond the muscular wall of the colon into the mesocolic fat, it becomes a pericolic abscess (Hughes, 1975). The abscess wall may incorporate any adjacent structure, small or large intestine, bladder, uterus, omentum, or parietal peritoneum. Resolution of the abscess is possible with appropriate antibiotic chemotherapy; however, the larger the abscess, the more likely it is to require drainage for complete resolution.

Drainage is usually spontaneous and back into the bowel lumen. The original inflammatory tract is often the line of least resistance. Pus may dissect along the bowel before returning to the lumen. If the original inflammatory tract from lumen to abscess remains, usually termed a communicating abscess, then an enteric fistula will form. More distant loops of intestine, particularly the mobile small intestine, may become incorporated into the abscess wall. Drainage can then occur into the ileum or jejunum, and if the original tract from colon to abscess remains intact, an ileocolic or jejunocolic fistula can result. Abscess may discharge into adjacent organs, such as the bladder, or through the abdominal wall. With each location there is the risk of fistula formation.

Evacuation into the peritoneal cavity will result in peritonitis. If the original tract from the colon to the abscess has sealed, then this noncommunicating peritonitis is readily managed with antibiotics and drainage (Hughes, 1975). A communicating peritonitis with ongoing fecal soilage usually requires more vigorous surgical management, with some procedure to resolve the perforation as well as to defunctionalize the distal colon.

Adequate drainage without fistula formation usually permits complete resolution of the abscess. In years gone by, abscess was a difficult diagnosis. It was simply one of several possible space-occupying lesions located in an area diagnostically difficult to approach. With the advent of the CAT scan and ultrasonography, there are now noninvasive and highly accurate tools to use in the identification of abscess. These modalities make it possible to follow the resolution of a collection and the identification of failures to respond. Failure of resolution of an abscess with appropriate antibiotic therapy, particularly in the face of clinical evidence of advancing toxicity, merits the consideration of immediate surgical intervention to effect drainage or resect the abscess.

Fistula

Fistula may form as a result of spontaneous or surgical drainage of a communicating abscess. Generally this is in a clinical setting and is an exacerbation of the diverticulitis with pain and fever. The fistula may also be the presenting event without the antecedent signs and symptoms of acute diverticulitis. This seems to be a matter of timing rather than of some intrinsic difference in the pathogenesis of each kind of fistula.

The most common clinically apparent fistulae are vesicocolic. The diverticulitis is often silent; the presentation is that of recurrent cystitis (Henderson & Small, 1969), and males are most often affected. The mechanism is related to the relatively motile segment of the pelvic sigmoid colon. When this short segment of the sigmoid becomes involved with diverticulitis, it is so positioned as to become adherent to the posterior wall of the bladder. A small connecting abscess evacuating through the wall of the bladder will create the fistula. Any substantial prior experience with diverticulitis in this segment would shorten the colon and prevent contact with the bladder wall. The lack of a past history of symptomatic inflammation is essential to the pathophysiology of the development of this fistula. Male predominance is explained by the protective cover which the uterus offers to the back of the bladder in females.

The clinical presentation is that of recurrent cystitis with dysuria and frequency of urination. Pneumaturia is a frequent finding in men but is rarely described in women. This is due to the fact that pneumaturia is observed but not felt. In the upright patient, the gas bubble in the bladder sits atop the urine and its passage follows the passage of urine (Henderson & Small, 1969). The urethra is no more perceptive than the anal canal (see Chapter 5), and liquid and gas "feel" the same to the mucosa. Males generally observe their urinary stream while females do not, and thus only men are aware that they are passing "air." Fortunately, as was mentioned, women have some protection from fistula in the first place.

Diagnosis can be difficult. Generally the pressures within the colon are higher than the intravesical pressure (Small & Smith, 1975). For this reason the presentation is usually that of a urinary tract abnormality. In the elderly male with a tendency for outlet obstruction as benign prostatic hypertrophy develops, passage of urine through the rectum can occur. Fistula is in the differential diagnosis of watery diarrhea.

Cystoscopy may show a patch of cystitis on the bladder wall, but only rarely will it visualize the opening of the fistulous tract. Cystograms with radiopaque media rarely visualize the tract. An approach from the bowel is similarly unrewarding. Barium does not regularly visualize the tract, and the tract opening is also not distinctive on sigmoidoscopy. An upright x-ray may show the air in the bladder, particularly if done immediately after a sigmoidoscopy. A high index of suspicion and pneumaturia are the two best clues to the diagnosis. Surgical resection is the only practical approach to management.

Fistula may form to the small intestine, either ileum or jejunum. Ileocolic fistula involving distal ileum are often completely silent and are incidental findings at a barium enema examination. As the entry of the fistulous tract creeps higher, malabsorption may become evident. Bypass of the receptors for B_{12} can eventually lead to megaloblastic anemia. Bypass of the receptors for bile acid resorption can spill bile acids into the colon which, when deconjugated by bacteria, results in diarrhea. Often medical management will suffice with appropriate replacement therapy and binding resins for bile acids. Should these fail, then there is an option for surgical resection. Diagnosis may be confusing, particularly with ileocolic fistula where differentiation from Crohn's disease is a concern.

Colocutaneous and colovaginal fistula are uncommon. With a colovaginal fistula, one is always concerned about carcinoma of the cervix as an etiology. Crohn's disease is also a consideration. Postirradiation colitis with fistula should be apparent from history.

Obstruction

Intestinal obstruction during an acute attack of diverticulitis may be due to adynamic ileus or to obstruction by an inflammatory mass (Hughes, 1975). In chronic disease, scarring and kinking of the lumen may produce partial or complete obstruction. The partial obstruction in this case may fluctuate as the inflammatory process waxes and wanes. Either kind of obstruction can involve the small or the large intestine. Complete obstruction is an emergency readily recognized in a patient with distention, vomiting, and air fluid levels in the bowel on upright x-ray of the abdomen. Peritoneal soiling with resultant adynamic ileus must be differentiated from obstruction by an inflammatory mass.

Obstruction without peritonitis should be managed conservatively, with the patient placed NPO to give bowel rest parenteral fluids administered to maintain hydration and electrolyte balance. The patient needs to be followed in a serial fashion, with the anticipation that the control of the inflammation will permit relief of the obstruction. Urgent surgery, particularly in the elderly, is always at the price of increased morbidity and mortality. Once the obstruction is relieved and the patient is stabilized, definitive evaluation for the possibility of surgical intervention is in order. The management of obstruction secondary to ileus associated with peritonitis has been discussed above.

RIGHT-SIDED DIVERTICULOSIS

Most of the discussion above concerning the pathologic physiology of the development of diverticula is based on change observed grossly and microscopically in the sigmoid and distal descending colon. Diverticula do occur on the right side of the colon and except for the final present. These are false diverticula without organized muscle layers in the wall. In many instances, only mucosal remnants will remain, and the wall of the cyst is made up of fibrous elements and inflammatory cells (Muhletaler, et al., 1981). The cysts contain gas, often also fluid or feces. Although adhesions may form to surrounding organs (Gallagher & Welch, 1979), many of these diverticula will remain quite mobile and can present in any part of the abdomen.

The mechanism of giant sigmoid diverticulum formation has been a hotbed of speculation without much consensus. In many patients these structures form after a long period of chronic diverticulitis. This could be a simple coincidence, since a large share of the patients have no antecedent clinical symptoms that would suggest diverticulitis yet present with giant diverticulum (Moss, 1975). A number of other theories are current, including intermittent obstruction of a diverticulum, and these have been reviewed by Muhletaler and colleagues (1981).

Clinical Presentation

Two clinical presentations are described (Moss, 1975). Some patients will present with pain, usually felt in the left lower quadrant, and nausea. There may be a history of rectal bleeding either bright red blood or melena. On physical examination there often is tenderness suggesting peritoneal irritation. A mass is commonly palpable and may have been noted by the patient. Often these are of impressive size. The second general pattern of presentation is that of a large abdominal mass, sometimes enlarging, at other times fluctuating in size, associated with little or no other abdominal symptomatology.

Diagnosis and Differential Diagnosis

The key diagnostic study is the plain film of the abdomen (Fig. 6–6). This will reveal a gas-filled cystic structure. Other imaging techniques can show this with even greater clarity but also at greater cost. A barium enema examination occasionally will identify a connection between the lumen and the diverticulum, and it can outline the mass lesion. The barium study can also confirm the presence of sigmoid diverticular disease as well.

The differential diagnosis includes a wide variety of gas-containing mass lesions in the abdomen (Table 6–2). Most may be differentiated in a relatively straightforward manner. Pancreatic and biliary cysts are readily diagnosed. Intestinal duplications tend to present in younger patients. Volvulus of segments of the large intestine (see below), pseudo-obstruction, and pneumatosis cystoides intestinalis can be more

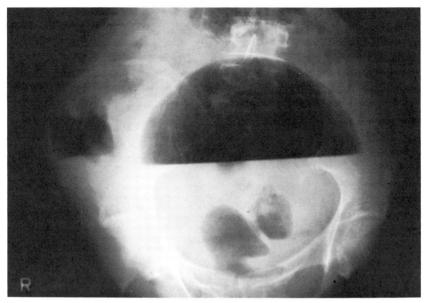

Figure 6–6. Radiograph showing the dilated air- and fluid-containing giant colonic diverticulum. (Courtesy of Dr. Peter Meyers.)

difficult to differentiate, but the acute presentation and the use of the newer imaging methods have simplified this small diagnostic dilemma. Sigmoid volvulus, also a problem of the elderly, is differentiated by fiberoptic endoscopy.

TABLE 6–2. Differential Diagnosis of "Air Cysts"* in the Abdomen

Mechanical obstruction	Diverticulosis
Sigmoid volvulus	Meckel's diverticulum
Colon volvulus	Giant duodenal diverticulum
Transverse colon volvulus	Acute gastric dilatation
Carcinoma of the colon	Biliary lesions
Functional obstruction	Cholecystenteric fistula
Pseudo-obstruction	Emphysematous cholecystitis
Drugs	Pancreatic pseudocysts, infected
Anticholinergic	Vesical lesions
Antiparkinsonian	Emphysematous cystitis
Megacolon (acquired)	Vesicoenteric fistula
Toxic megacolon	Lipoma
Pneumatosis cystoides	Intraabdominal abscess
Giant diverticulum	

*Radiological "air cysts" occur in the abdominal cavity. These radiolucent lesions are associated with many and varied diagnoses.

Management

Treatment is surgical resection of the diverticulum and, if possible, restoration of colon continuity (Gallagher & Welch, 1979). The operation is rarely an emergency, and there is time to prepare the patient for surgery. The general condition of the elderly patient is often the determinant of the management of this nonemergent problem.

VOLVULUS OF THE COLON

Volvulus can occur in any segment of the colon with a mesentery long enough to permit the segment to twist. The sigmoid colon generally has that degree of mobility. As a normal anatomical variant, many people have an extraordinary mobility of the cecum which permits it to twist. Generally more than unusual mobility is required to precipitate cecal volvulus, although the associated problems are varied. These include prior abdominal surgery, particularly appendectomy, distal colon obstruction, or serious intercurrent medical illness. Anatomical variants in the transverse colon can also afford a mesentery long enough to produce a twist, but this is very uncommon. Here also some additional feature, such as an adhesion or distal obstruction, is a necessary component of the torsion (Wertkin & Aufses, 1978).

Volvulus of the colon is a common cause of intestinal obstruction, and it has a curious and poorly understood geographical variability. In the United States, the accepted figure is 3 to 5 per cent of intestinal obstruction caused by volvulus of the colon (Wertkin & Aufses, 1978). Similar figures for Scandinavia and the Soviet Union, particularly the Soviet Baltic states are 30 to 50 per cent (Bruusgaard, 1947). Sigmoid volvulus is a disease of elderly men. The average age of occurrence is in the high 60's and there are few cases under age 55. Cecal volvulus is a disease predominantly of older women with the average age of onset being 53. Transverse colon volvulus occurs in a younger age group. There is no acceptable explanation for the reported sex, geographical, and age distributions (Wertkin & Aufses, 1978).

Sigmoid Volvulus

This is a chronic, recurrent (if not definitively treated) disease of high mortality. Mortality rates of 20 per cent and higher are reported, and this increases with recurrent attacks. The age of the patient and the likelihood of complicating intercurrent disease undoubtedly are factors in this high mortality (Hines, et al., 1967).

Pathology and Pathologic Physiology

Clockwise torsion of 180° is considered a physiological volvulus. A 180° counterclockwise twist is a step toward volvulus but is tolerated. A 360° counterclockwise twist produces a closed loop obstruction in the sigmoid colon. This twist may produce obstruction alone or with strangulation. Tension in the closed loop and the tightness of the twist are factors in the development of strangulation (Bruusgaard, 1947). No particular features seem to stand out as precipitants of the volvulus. The pathologic findings are those of any closed loop obstruction and vary with the duration of the problem.

Clinical Presentation

The initial symptoms are those of crampy abdominal pain and distention. Often there is a history of recurrent bouts of pain which may be due to incomplete torsion and spontaneous detorsion of the sigmoid loop over months or years before volvulus completes a closed loop obstruction. For this reason patients may not recognize the gravity of the initial symptoms and do not present to the physician until distant signs of intestinal obstruction emerge. These more distant signs are gradual in development. There is the onset of nausea and vomiting which with time will become feculent. Once the rectum and the bit of sigmoid distal to the obstruction has emptied—and this may take the form of diarrhea—constipation will intervene. As the vascular supply to the loop is compromised, attention returns to the lower abdomen with increasing pain and systemic toxicity.

Physical findings are tenderness and a mass in the lower abdomen. As the obstruction progresses, there may be visible peristalsis. The rectum is usually empty. Occasionally there is a small amount of gross rectal bleeding. As tension builds in the closed loop peritoneal, signs will become apparent. If neglected, perforation will develop with accompanying rigid abdomen. Chills, fever, and tachycardia all point toward abdominal catastrophe.

Laboratory studies early on will show evidence of dehydration and, as the obstruction progresses, elevation in the white count and the percentage of polymorphonuclear cells.

Diagnosis and Differential Diagnosis

The plain film of the abdomen shows the characteristic gas-distended loop of bowel in the lower abdomen (Fig. 6–7). Traditionally a barium enema was the next step. One looked for a characteristic "bird beak" configuration as the barium column reached the tapering point of obstruction at the twist (Fig. 6–8) (Glick & Laufer, 1988). A more direct approach using the fiberoptic sigmoidoscope is currently the

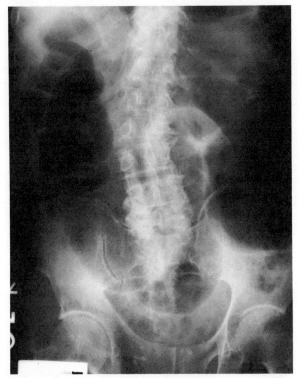

Figure 6–7. Radiograph showing the characteristic distended loop of gas-filled bowel found in patients with sigmoid volvulus. Compare this with Figure 6–6. (Courtesy of Dr. Peter Meyers.)

diagnostic tool of choice. Endoscopically one sees only the tapering obstruction but a careful advance of the scope achieves a high percentage of nonoperative reductions of the volvulus to confirm the diagnosis.

Management

If there is no clinical evidence of perforation, then endoscopic reduction should be attempted. Failure to reduce the volvulus obligates emergency surgery. If the reduction is successful, there remains a bit of a dilemma concerning further management. In an elderly patient or in anyone compromised by other medical problems that make even elective surgery an unacceptable hazard, one enters a period of sensitized waiting. The reported recurrence rates are as high as 40 per cent. The patient and/or the caregiver need to share in the understanding of the serious hazards of a recurrence. With intact bowel, recurrence carries a mortality rate greater than 10 per cent; with gangrene of the bowel, it is 50 per cent. Early intervention is essential.

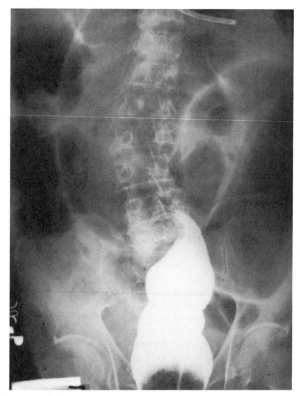

Figure 6–8. Radiograph showing a barium enema in the patient illustrated in Figure 6–7 with sigmoid volvulus. The barium column tapers to form the characteristic bird beak appearance that is diagnostic of the twisted bowel. A similar appearance can be seen in some cases of cecal volvulus. (Courtesy of Dr. Peter Meyers.)

If the reduction is successful and the patient's condition will permit safe elective surgery, then definitive repair should be carried out during that hospitalization (Thayer & Denucci, 1988a). Any suggestion of gangrene requires immediate surgery.

Cecal Volvulus

While cecal volvulus has been characterized as a problem of elderly women, men also are at risk. The sex ratio only slightly favors women. Age may be much less a factor than has been thought (O'Mara, et al., 1980). Cecal volvulus is not common and accounts for only one per cent of intestinal obstructions (O'Mara, et al., 1980). Like sigmoid volvulus it has a lethal potential, with mortality rates in older series varying from 30 to 60 per cent (Hendrick, 1964). Mortality in more recent series is the same as in sigmoid volvulus (O'Mara, et al., 1980).

Pathology and Pathologic Physiology

The cecum ordinarily hangs free in the peritoneal cavity. To twist enough to produce a closed loop obstruction, it must be hypermotile. Hypermotility is a normal variant that occurs in up to 25 per cent of people (Hendrick, 1964). Usually there is some second feature that in some way is a coprecipitant of the problem. Commonly there is a history of prior abdominal surgery to raise the specter of an adhesion creating a fixed point around which the cecum twists. Recent surgery (within days), acute medical problems, and the early postpartum state have also been implicated by association. For the latter, mechanisms are not clear.

The findings at surgery are those of a closed loop obstruction. Viewed from the front, the twist is a clockwise turn winding the distal ileum and the ascending colon to produce the closed loop.

Clinical Presentation

Hinshaw and colleagues (1959) distinguish three clinical presentations, and their classification has stood the test of time. A sudden twist will produce an acute fulminating presentation, and presumably there is early compromise of the circulation. Pain develops rapidly, and there is early evidence of peritoneal irritation.

A second presentation is acute but obstructive rather than ischemic in its symptomatology. One finds a huge gas-filled loop of bowel. The symptomatology is acute and generally very nonspecific early in the course. There may be some right lower quadrant discomfort, but it is often not severe enough to attract attention until vomiting begins. There will be modest abdominal distention, and, if left to progress, peritoneal signs will develop.

The third variety is an intermittent obstruction and can be difficult to diagnose unless studies coincide with the torsion.

Diagnosis and Differential Diagnosis

Plain film of the abdomen is again the indicator of the diagnosis. Newer imaging techniques are even more adept at identifying the dilated gas-filled cecum. A barium enema will show the classic "bird beak" sign in many; in others it will show a cut off in the column of barium. There should be radiological evidence of small bowel obstruction.

Cecal volvulus is in the differential diagnosis of intestinal obstruction. When a gas-filled cecum can be identified, the differential diagnosis is limited to those few lesions that present the radiological appearance of a gas cyst. These include sigmoid volvulus, giant sigmoid diverticulum, intestinal duplications, gas-containing abscesses and pseudo-obstruction, plus a host of very rare lesions.

Management

The management of cecal obstruction is surgical. Attempts at reduction of the volvulus by enema or with the colonoscope are not thought to be safe or, for that matter, very effective. Timely surgery that anticipates dead bowel will lower the mortality.

Volvulus of the Transverse Colon

This is a rare lesion, and it usually involves the younger patient. Diagnosis and management are much the same as for cecal volvulus, with the exception that there is a possible role for colonoscopy in reduction of the volvulus (Gumbs, et al., 1983).

MEGACOLON

Megacolon and pseudo-obstruction of the colon are variously combined and separated in the literature. Here they will be treated as separate entities, with megacolon defined as chronic dilatation of the colon without intervening periods of normal colonic appearance and function, and pseudo-obstruction as acute dilatation but with reversion of the colon to normal appearances during remission. Both in fact are variants of adynamic ileus. The megasigmoid syndrome is a recognized variant common in patients with neuropsychiatric problems. Toxic megacolon will be discussed in the section on chronic ulcerative colitis.

Pathology and Pathologic Physiology

There are several widely differing mechanisms that result in acquired megacolon. The exotic aganglionosis secondary to trypanosome infection is not an aging problem (Todd, 1971). The aganglionosis secondary to chronic use of anthraquinone laxatives certainly can account for some (but not all) cases of acquired megacolon in the elderly (Smith, 1968). The remaining cases are found in institutionalized patients in either nursing homes or psychiatric facilities. The usual explanation is that chronic neglect of bowel function, with resultant constipation that causes gradual enlargement of the colon full of hard, dry, retained feces. A second, possibly necessary, factor is a primary or degenerative muscle disorder that permits the colonic dilatation (Todd, 1971). In the elderly a degenerative disorder would be suspect.

Patients with severe constipation but intact musculature do not necessarily develop dilatation. Pathologic changes in the colon are not distinctive.

Clinical Presentation

The clinical presentation is that of abdominal distention coupled with diarrhea. Fecal incontinence is also a common occurrence. While the underlying problem is a variety of constipation, the impacted fecal mass often produces enough irritation to cause diarrhea around the impactions. Incontinence in some is related to the underlying disease and in others to the loss of sensitivity and discrimination in the overloaded rectum.

Diagnosis

The diagnosis is largely one of exclusion of other possible etiologies of a chronic partial obstruction. The large feces-filled colon poses some technical hindrance to diagnosis, but once the colon is cleansed, a barium enema and colonoscopy will rule out most confusing diagnoses.

Management

There is little or nothing that can be done concerning the underlying lesion. There is a great deal to be done in terms of keeping the bowel clean. This needs to be individualized to the patient's tolerance and to the setting, which for many patients will be institutional care. A large feces-filled colon is susceptible to volvulus. Careful cleansing can remove this risk.

PSEUDO-OBSTRUCTION

Pseudo-obstruction can involve any level of the colon and the urinary tract as well (see Chapter 3). A clinical presentation limited to the colon is not uncommon. Massive acute dilatation of the colon without evidence of an organic obstructing lesion is observed in a variety of settings. The primary form is ascribed to neuromuscular abnormalities that are not yet well characterized. It has no particular predilection for the elderly. Secondary forms (see Table 3–3) do include a number of problems that are age related.

Pathology and Pathologic Physiology

The clinical problem is that of adynamic ileus. This may involve the entire colon or a segment alone. There is frequently localization in the cecum and in the right colon. Acute involvement of the cecum can be complicated by cecal rupture (Thayer & Denucci, 1988b). Without rupture, pathologic changes are limited to massive distention of the colonic segment. Mechanisms vary with the underlying problem (see Table 3–3).

Clinical Presentation

The patient appears distended, but short of catastrophic complication, there are few symptoms. Depending largely on the duration of the attack there may be nausea and vomiting. When colonic pseudo-obstruction is associated with involvement in the small intestine, it is difficult to ascribe the origin of the symptoms. When the colon alone is involved, symptomatology is mild (Faulk, et al., 1978). There is abdominal tenderness, and if this localizes, then there is concern about impending perforation. Cecal perforation will lead to presentation as an acute abdomen.

Diagnosis and Differential Diagnosis

A plain film of the abdomen is the first step in diagnosis. Distended gas-filled loops of colon lead to a modest differential (Table 6–2). Organic obstruction by tumor, volvulus, or ischemia are pressing diagnoses. Toxic megacolon also requires immediate assessment. Endoscopy with the colonoscope or fiberoptic sigmoidoscope is emerging as a direct solution to the problem. In the hugely distended colon of pseudo-obstruction, preparation, or the lack of it, is not often a problem.

Management

Definitive management of pseudo-obstruction rests with control of the underlying condition that has predisposed to its occurrence. There is an immediate concern for the comfort of the patient and for the prevention of perforation. Patients should be placed NPO and the intravenous route used to maintain fluid and electrolyte balance. Predisposing drugs that can be stopped or substituted should be changed. Colonoscopic decompression can gain needed time to permit spontaneous return of bowel function (Strodel, et al., 1983). Perforation or impending perforation requires surgical decompression.

CHRONIC ULCERATIVE COLITIS

Idiopathic inflammatory bowel disease includes three separate entities: chronic ulcerative colitis, ulcerative proctitis, and Crohn's disease. While these three diseases share many elements in terms of epidemiology, presentation, and management, each behaves in a clinically distinct fashion. The intestinal manifestations of chronic ulcerative colitis and ulcerative proctitis are confined to the colon, but Crohn's disease may involve any level of the digestive tube.

Pathology and Pathologic Physiology

Chronic ulcerative colitis is a chronic, usually recurrent although sometimes continuous, inflammatory disease of the mucosa of the colon. The inflammation characteristically results in mucosal ulceration (Table 6–3). The involvement usually begins in the rectum and sigmoid and may remain confined to the distal colon or may progressively involve the entire colon. Some patients start with total involvement. A minimal involvement of the terminal ileus—termed backwash ileitis—is described. In active colitis the involved mucosa has a relatively featureless granular appearance, and there is often evidence of hemorrhage. Ulcerations are usually but not invariably present; these penetrate only the thickness of the mucosa and may undermine adjacent intact mucosa. This overlying mucosa may become edematous and swollen with inflammatory cells to form a pseudopolyp. Intact mucosa is friable and will bleed with any minor trauma. With severe disease the inflammatory process can extend more deeply into the muscular wall. Involvement tends to be contiguous without intervening normal areas. In remission the mucosal ulcers are healed, and the mucosa itself loses its friability.

TABLE 6–3. Pathologic Features of Crohn's Disease and Ulcerative Colitis

	CROHN'S DISEASE	ULCERATIVE COLITIS
Gross Features		
Anal and perianal lesions	Major and common	Minor and uncommon
Bowel wall	Thickened	Normal to slight increase
Strictures	Common	Uncommon
Fistulas	Common	Rare
Pseudopolyps	Rare	Common
Ulcers	Fissure	Punctate to troughlike
Distribution	More proximal	More distal
Continuity	Often "skip" areas	Always contiguous
Toxic megacolon	Uncommon	More common
Carcinoma	Rare	Increased
Microscopic Features		
Primary impact	Submucosa	Mucosa
Type of reaction	Productive	Exudative
Lymphoreticular hyperplasia	Marked and transmural	Minimal and superficial
Granulomas	40 to 80%	Occasional
Crypt abscesses	Occasional	Usual
Vascular ectasia and edema	Marked	Related to acute inflammation
Epithelial regeneration	Rare	Common

From Watson, D. W.: The problem of chronic inflammatory bowel disease. Calif Med 117:25, 1972. Reprinted by permission of the Western Journal of Medicine (formerly California Medicine).

In addition, an assortment of extraintestinal manifestations (listed in Table 6–4) of chronic ulcerative colitis are variable in occurrence. Some of these, such as nephrolithiasis and pericholangitis, are secondary complications with a reasonable explanation for the mechanism. Others, particularly the joint, skin, and eye lesions, have no clear-cut mechanism and may be related to the primary cause of the colitis.

The cause of chronic ulcerative colitis remains unknown. A great deal of study devoted to the disease's epidemiology and to altered immune relationships has produced no more than tantalizing hints concerning the underlying mechanism. While chronic ulcerative colitis is found worldwide, there are significant geographical variations in incidence and prevalence. It seems to occur more commonly in whites than in blacks, in Jews than in Gentiles, in urban settings than in rural ones, and in families with an affected member. The peak age incidence for chronic ulcerative colitis is between 15 and 20 years. More pertinent to this text, there is a late peak of occurrence in the 55 to 60-year old group. This is a small percentage of chronic ulcerative colitis patients but not a rare occurrence (Mendeloff, 1980). Several explanations have been offered for this late peak of occurrence. It may be that this represents a second disease entity, but there is nothing concrete to support this suggestion. Another possibility, suggested by Rogers and colleagues (1971) is that this represents the emergence of mesenteric vascular insufficiency, which interacts with the unknown primary factor to produce colitis.

There has been a clear demonstration that lymphocytes from patients with chronic ulcerative colitis are cytotoxic for colon epithelial cells. Anticolon antibodies are present in many patients. Many other abnormalities of the immune system are described. All of these studies suggest that there is some immune mechanism involved in the continuing damage of the mucosa, but none identify what it is that initiates the process.

TABLE 6–4. Extraintestinal Manifestations of Inflammatory Bowel Diseases

Skin and mucous membrane	Musculoskeletal
Erythema nodosum	Arthritis of extremities
Pyoderma gangrenosum	Sacroiliitis
Oral aphthous ulcer	Ankylosing spondylitis
	Clubbing of the fingers
Eye	**Liver and biliary tract**
Iritis	Pericholangitis
Conjunctivitis	Fatty liver
Episcleritis	Sclerosing cholangitis
	Kidney
	Nephrolithiasis
	Hydronephrosis

Clinical Presentation

The hallmarks of chronic ulcerative colitis are diarrhea and rectal bleeding, ranging in severity from slight loosening of stools with occult blood present to bloody dysentery. The severity of the symptomatology seems roughly related to the extent of the colonic involvement. Involvement of the rectum when severe produces tenesmus. Cramping abdominal pain at the time of bowel movements is a common complaint. Gross blood may be mixed with the stool or streaked on the outside of the fecal pellet.

Physical findings may be very minor. Slight abdominal tenderness may be all that one can demonstrate in mild attacks. As the severity of the attack progresses, so does the occurrence of physical findings—tachycardia, pallor, abdominal distention, and ultimately peritoneal signs can be found as severity progresses. Extraintestinal manifestations (Table 6–4) may precede or accompany the acute attack. While most extraintestinal manifestations will improve with remission, some will progress.

As the name implies, the disease is chronic. In some patients this takes the form of remissions and exacerbations. The remissions may be so complete that the bowel appears normal. In other patients the disease remains continuously active, although the level of activity may fluctuate widely. The outcome of any particular attack is related more closely to the severity of that attack than to any other feature (Edwards & Truelove, 1963). Meaningful clinical criteria to grade the severity of an attack were described by Edwards and Truelove (1963) and have been revised and sharpened since then (Goodman & Sparberg, 1978; Cello, 1983; Kirsner & Shorter, 1988). Attacks are graded as mild, moderate, and severe.

Mild disease is characterized by three or fewer bowel movements daily with little or no gross blood, no anemia, no fever, and no resting tachycardia. Criteria for moderate disease include four to ten stools daily with gross blood, anemia with a hemoglobin of 11.5 gm or more, and resting tachycardia. Fever is present, but it may be low grade. Weight loss is less than 10 per cent of pre-illness weight. Patients with severe attacks have ten or more stools daily, all with gross blood, abdominal cramps, and vomiting. Weight loss exceeds 10 per cent of their stable weight. Anemia with hemoglobin below 11.5 gm, fever of 100°F (37.8°C) or more, hypoalbuminemia, and an elevated sedimentation rate of at least 30 mm/hr are other signs of severe attack (Edwards & Truelove, 1963; Kirsner & Shorter, 1988).

As with any such classification, the strength of any particular criterion is subject to modification by good clinical judgment. This is particularly true in the elderly, who may have already compromised much of their physiological reserve with other medical problems or with their therapy. The goal is to judge the severity of the attack with objective criteria; the system works quite well in younger patients and early in the course of the disease. As patients' problems become chronic and are compounded by several simultaneous disease processes, grading is not so cleanly done.

Diagnosis and Differential Diagnosis

With the initial attack it is possible to have a strong clinical suspicion concerning the diagnosis, but endoscopy, biopsy, and radiological examination are usually required to confirm the diagnosis. Even with the completion of all studies, there will still remain 20 per cent of cases in whom the differentiation of chronic ulcerative colitis from Crohn's colitis is in question (Kirsner & Shorter, 1988).

Endoscopy

Endoscopic examination, usually beginning with the fiberoptic sigmoidoscope, a rigid sigmoidoscope, or a proctoscope, should be attempted on the unprepared rectum. In a patient with diarrhea, the rectum after a bowel movement will often be clean enough to permit examination. A later follow-up complete sigmoidoscopy with an adequately prepared sigmoidoscopic examination is mandatory, but the initial look is best performed on a rectum undamaged by enema. This simple procedure can be done in the office at the time of the initial visit to permit initiation of therapy without delay after the diagnosis has been confirmed.

The mucosa will appear granular, often the phrase "a ground glass appearance" is used. In normals the mucosa is shiny and transparent, and the underlying vascular pattern is readily visible through it. When the mucosa is inflamed in colitis, edema develops and breaks up the light reflection from the no longer smooth surface, hence the granular or ground glass appearance. This also affects the transparency of the mucosa, and the underlying vascular pattern is no longer clearly visible. The second feature of colitic mucosa is friability. The inflamed mucosa is extraordinarily fragile, and the tip of the endoscope or a swab will produce bleeding. Hemorrhage and ulceration may or may not be present. The ulcers when present are shallow, superficial lesions with exudate in the base. Mucus secretion is stimulated, and in some patients large amounts of thick mucus will be present. Pseudopolyps may be seen. These inflamed remnants of mucosa are adjacent to ulcerated areas.

In chronic continuous cases or after multiple recurrences, the mucosa may become scarred and may appear featureless, pink, and with no visible vascular pattern. As healing progresses the loss of friability is usually the first notable change. Involvement usually begins in the rectum. In fact, if the rectum is spared (and this does occasionally occur in chronic ulcerative colitis), it is cause to question the diagnosis. Rectal biopsy using the small clamshell forceps will permit confirmation of the inflammation and will provide a permanent record of the lesion. These tiny forceps are safe but allow only mucosal biopsies.

Anoscopy, while probably not essential, is a valuable adjunct to the examination. In patients with rectal pain, narrowing of the stools, and decrease in stool caliber, anoscopy is mandatory. Many endoscopists believe that they get an acceptable view of the anal canal by slow withdrawal of the sigmoidoscope, but the view is never so clear as it is with carefully done anoscopy. When cultures are desired (and the problem of differentiation of *Campylobacter jejuni*, *Clostridium difficile*, and gonococcal infection is ever with us), they are better taken with an anoscope than through a fiberoptic endoscope.

Colonoscopy is not usually the first endoscopic procedure. It is important in determination of the extent of involvement and the activity of the disease. The patient must be able to tolerate the lavage necessary to cleanse the colon. Often one must wait until the acute attack has begun to moderate before attempting colonoscopy. In the follow-up of patients with chronic disease, colonoscopy is often the only diagnostic tool that will permit assessment of the activity of the disease process. It is essential in the evaluation of the mucosa for signs of neoplastic change. The procedure is in the hands of trained specialists.

Radiography

The barium enema x-ray examination neither replaces nor is replaced by, endoscopy. They are complementary techniques for evaluation of the colon in inflammatory bowel disease. The barium enema gives an excellent idea of the extent of disease and the extent of shortening that may have occurred in the colon. It is not as sensitive in the evaluation of the state of the mucosa.

Differential Diagnosis

The initial problem is to rule out specific forms of inflammatory bowel disease. Many of these can be identical in appearance grossly, radiologically, and microscopically, and only demonstration of the infecting organism can make the diagnosis. Table 6–5 lists organisms capable of causing proctocolitis. Of this group *Campylobacter*, gonococci, and *C. difficile* toxin are the most common offenders. The appropriate use of smear, culture, and serology is the only solution to the diagnosis.

A variety of drug-induced changes can occur in the colon and must

TABLE 6–5. Etiological Agents in Infectious Proctocolitis

Bacteria	Fungi
Campylobacter jejuni	*Candida albicans*
Gonococci	
Salmonella sp.	**Virus**
Shigella sp.	Herpes simplex
Vibrio parahaemolyticus	
Escherichia coli	**Protozoa**
Yersinia sp.	*Cryptosporidium*
	Entamoeba histolytica
Bacteria Toxins	*Dientamoeba fragilis*
Clostridium difficile	
Staphylococcal enterotoxin	

be considered in diagnosis. Because of the frequency with which the elderly take drugs, they are at unusual risk. Many of the cathartics will, with prolonged use, produce changes in the colon that can mimic some stages of chronic ulcerative colitis. Gold salts and methyldopa can also be responsible for changes.

Another problem of the elderly is ischemic colitis. Diarrhea, ulceration, pain, and bleeding are all features of ischemic colitis and can overlap the presentation of chronic ulcerative colitis. As mentioned above, there is speculation that the late age peak in chronic ulcerative colitis cases may in fact represent an interaction between a compromised vascular supply and the primary mechanism for chronic ulcerative colitis.

The largest part of the problem of differential diagnosis is distinguishing ulcerative colitis from Crohn's colitis. These entities will be discussed further on in this chapter.

Management

The goal of management of chronic ulcerative colitis is the induction and maintenance of a remission. The approach to mild, moderate, and severe disease differs. The treatment of the elderly does not differ qualitatively from the treatment of younger patients. Quantitatively, disease, with its onset in the elderly, seems more aggressive, and because of this and the frequency with which other complicating diseases occur, more older patients fall into the moderate and severe categories. Worse yet the mortality rate of elderly patients with severe disease is higher than in younger patients with severe disease (Cello, 1983).

Mild Disease

Patients with mild chronic ulcerative colitis may be treated as outpatients. Sulfasalazine is the mainstay of drug therapy; it is split in the colon by bacterial action to produce sulfapyridine and 5-aminosali-cylic acid. The sulfapyridine has an antimicrobial action and is handled by the body as any other absorbable sulfonamide. Sensitivity to sulfa drugs is a contraindication to the use of sulfasalazine. The 5-aminosal-icylic acid is an active agent in the colon in the treatment of chronic ulcerative colitis. A number of rectal and oral preparations of 5-aminosalicylic acid are under study.

The dose should be the smallest that seems to be effective and will vary from patient to patient. The range of dosage is 2 to 4 gm daily, but an occasional patient will require 6 or 8 gm daily to achieve an effect. Higher dosages are associated with substantial increases in drug reactions. Drug reactions seem to take two forms. The first is a matter of irritation of the upper digestive tract. The use of enteric-coated tablets and a 1.5 or 2 gm daily starting dose, with an increase of 0.5 gm daily until the full dose is reached, will avoid many irritative side effects for which the elderly are especially prone. True sensitivity to the drug also occurs with skin rash, hemolysis, and hepatitis. There are many other less common reactions. The drug may interfere with folic acid absorption and supplementation may be necessary.

Antidiarrheal medication is not necessary in mild disease. Patients should be encouraged to eat the most nutritious diet that they can tolerate. It is wise to restrict milk products because of lactase deficiency, and during the acute attack, bulking agents are probably not in order. Common sense should prompt patients to avoid foods that cause an idiosyncratic reaction, but often this takes a timely reminder from the physician. The caregivers for elderly patients often need to be reassured that exotic supplements and diets are not necessary or desirable.

In the patient with severe rectal pain and tenesmus, a steroid enema or foam application may help to control these bothersome symptoms. Steroid enemas are also useful in patients who are sensitive to sulfasalazine.

Moderate Disease

Elderly patients with moderate disease require hospitalization. Treatment with sulfasalazine should be started as for mild disease. In addition, prednisone in doses of 40 mg orally daily should be started. If there is not a prompt response, the dose can be raised to 60 mg daily, or parenteral steroids may be given. Starting a course of steroids obligates the patient to four to six weeks of therapy followed by another four weeks of slow taper of the steroids. This is a dosage that will produce side effects.

During the initial days of hospitalization the patient may require intravenous fluids and electrolytes. If the patient is willing to eat, then this should be encouraged. High protein supplements are a mainstay of the early days of therapy. The anemia warrants iron therapy. Antidiarrheal agents should be avoided, as these may predispose to the development of toxic megacolon.

Failure to attain a remission can take several different clinical expressions. At any point the attack of chronic ulcerative colitis may worsen, and moderate disease may become severe disease. Generally this means that surgical intervention and colectomy are called for. In a few cases there will simply be no change or improvement. This too warrants surgical consultation. To persist with ineffective medical therapy in the face of unimproved moderate disease simply adds to the risk of the inevitable surgery.

The real medical problem rests with the patient who improves but fails to remit completely or who is unable to sustain a remission as the steroids are tapered. One is left with chronic steroid administration and, depending on the dosage, the gradual emergence of side effects. In the elderly patient already osteoporotic, the emergence of complications may not be so gradual. The steroids also complicate the management of hypertension and diabetes so prevalent in the older patient. The first strategy in this setting is to get the steroid dosage as low as possible by starting at a steroid dose that controls the symptoms. The taper from this dose must be ultra slow and in increments that, from the pharmacological standpoint, seem trivial, particularly as the taper approaches the lower end of the scale. At the lowest dose that one can achieve without recurrence, it is often worth trying to advance the sulfasalazine dose, but again slowly. If the patient tolerates an increase in sulfasalazine, then further taper of the steroids is in order. If taper of the steroids is arrested at a maintenance dose that is still unacceptably high, it is possible to get a steroid sparing effect with simultaneous administration of immunosuppressive drugs. Azathioprine and 6-mercaptopurine are the drugs used. Unfortunately these potent drugs have serious side effects. In the elderly patient whom you most want to wean to a lower steroid dose, immunosuppressives are often poorly tolerated. Geriatric patients are started on half of the usual doses of immunosuppressives, and the dosage is gradually increased with careful follow-up for toxicity and side effects (Skarin, 1985). When the tolerable dose of immunosuppressive is reached, then ultra slow taper of the steroids can again be tried. It takes a patient physician and an insightful patient to succeed.

Those patients who do achieve remission and who are taken off steroids should be maintained on sulfasalazine. This drug is effective in the maintenance of remissions (Summers, et al., 1979).

Severe Disease

These patients need to be hospitalized and to be seen and followed by the surgeon as well as by the internist. Intravenous steroids in doses equivalent to 200 to 300 mg of hydrocortisone daily are started. Invasive studies are restricted to limited sigmoidoscopy, and x-rays are limited to plain films. The risk of toxic megacolon is high, and therefore barium enema, preparation for endoscopy, endoscopy, or antidiarrheals, all known precipitants of megacolon, must be avoided. Fluid and electrolyte balance is maintained intravenously, and for at least the first several days, the patient's oral intake is limited to clear liquids. If there is any suggestion clinically or on the plain x-rays of the abdomen that toxic megacolon is imminent, then an antibiotic regimen should be started. This means parenteral administration of antibiotics selected to deal with contamination by mixed flora from the colon. Failure to respond or worsening within 24 to 48 hours should prompt surgical intervention.

Complications and Extraintestinal Manifestations

Extraintestinal manifestations may well be intrinsic components of the disease, but from the standpoint of management they are viewed as complications. In addition to the extraintestinal manifestations listed in Table 6–4, other complications include toxic megacolon, stricture of the colon, carcinoma of the colon, perforation of the colon, hemorrhage, amyloidosis, and thromboembolism.

Skin Lesions

Erythema nodosum is the most common skin lesion associated with chronic ulcerative colitis. It tends to come and go with the activity of the intestinal disease. Pyoderma gangrenosum is a much less common problem. These necrotizing ulcers, found most often on the legs, tend to be associated with severe chronic ulcerative colitis and are related to the activity of the intestinal disease. Occasionally the pyoderma can be severe enough to cause amputation or life-threatening infectious complications (Kern, 1980).

Mucous Membrane Lesions

Aphthous ulcer is a common finding during acute attacks. It requires only local symptomatic treatment (Edwards & Truelove, 1964).

Eye Lesions

Eye lesions tend to occur in patients who have active intestinal disease and other extraintestinal manifestations. They will improve as the colon improves or with its surgical removal. Consultation with an ophthalmologist is always in order. Although it is uncommon, corneal ulceration can become so severe as to threaten vision (Kern, 1980).

Bone and Joint Lesions

Arthralgia is very common during acute attacks of chronic ulcerative colitis. Objective evidence of arthritis is much less common, but it is not rare. Colitic arthritis is usually monoarticular and involves large joints such as the knee or ankle. The character of the joint inflammation resembles rheumatoid arthritis, but the distribution differs. There are no permanent sequelae. A few patients will have migratory polyarthritis. The joint inflammation tends to come on with an acute attack of colitis and will improve as the colon responds to treatment. Anti-inflammatory agents and physical therapy can help to make the patient comfortable (Kern, 1980).

Ankylosing spondylitis and sacroiliitis are much more common in patients with chronic ulcerative colitis than in the general population, but these seem to be associated diseases rather than complications of the colitis. Activity and progression of the spinal disease are not necessarily related to activity of the colitis; spinal disease may long precede the development of chronic ulcerative colitis (Kern, 1980).

Hepatobiliary Lesions

Fatty infiltration of the liver is very common in chronic ulcerative colitis, but it does not seem to be of clinical significance. Pericholangitis, while it is very common, does in a few cases progress to cirrhosis. While the etiology is not clear, it does seem to be associated with active colitis. Sclerosing cholangitis is a much less common and much more serious companion of chronic ulcerative colitis; however, this may well be an associated disease rather than a complication. The only definitive therapy is a liver transplant, but this is currently not available to the geriatric age group. Chronic active hepatitis is also an associated problem, but it is not common in the elderly with chronic ulcerative colitis.

Renal Disease

Renal stones are more common in chronic ulcerative colitis patients than in the general population, but the mechanism, unlike that in Crohn's disease involving ileum, is not at all clear.

Toxic Megacolon

Acute toxic megacolon is a complication of severe active colitis. Usually (but not invariably) it involves the entire colon. Megacolon affecting only segments of the colon is described, as is megacolon in other varieties of colitis. Megacolon is suspect when the diameter of the transverse colon on a supine plain film of the abdomen exceeds 6 cm. Toxic megacolon is suspect in a patient with chronic ulcerative colitis who has this dilatation associated with fever, tachycardia, abdominal pain, and distention (Cello, 1983).

The affected colon is the site of widespread ulceration and inflammation that extends to involve deeper layers of the colon wall. The musculature is paralyzed and distended until the wall of the colon is paper thin. The proximate cause of the syndrome is not clear. Prior barium enema, the administration of opiate antidiarrheal or analgesics, the use of anticholinergics, and hypokalemia are all well-known antecedents to the syndrome, but while these agents are used on, or occur in, many patients with chronic ulcerative colitis, only a few develop toxic megacolon (Edwards & Truelove, 1964; Cello, 1983).

The clinical appearance is as described above. These patients are desperately ill; they are febrile, distended, dehydrated, and weak. If diarrhea has been present, it may slow or cease. Physical examination will confirm the diffuse distention as gas, the bowel sounds are diminished or absent, and there is abdominal pain. Laboratory studies will show the anemia and hypoalbuminemia associated with the chronic ulcerative colitis and substantial leucocytosis as well. A supine plain film of the abdomen will show distention of the colon, usually the transverse colon in this view. There may be gas in the small intestine as well. This is the setting for colon perforation, and additional x-ray views must be taken to look for free air.

The findings listed above make the diagnosis, except in that infrequent case in which the toxic megacolon is the initial event ushering in the chronic ulcerative colitis. Where there is no prior diagnosis, a cautious, limited sigmoidoscopy may be required to confirm the diagnosis.

Management is in intensive care and must be individualized to the patient. Fluids and electrolytes, particularly potassium, must be calculated. In the elderly patient the margin between over treatment and under treatment is narrow; cardiovascular disease only exacerbates the problem. The patient should be NPO and on nasogastric suction. Steroids are given in daily heroic doses, 100 to 200 mg of prednisone administered parenterally. Many of these patients are either already on steroids for their chronic ulcerative colitis or have had steroid treatment in the past and may have residual suppression of the adrenals. Even in the absence of free air, broad spectrum antibiotics are in order.

In addition to the monitoring expected in the ICU, there need to be daily plain films of the abdomen. The abdomen should be carefully marked to facilitate repeated measurements of the girth. These two studies offer the best guide to improvement or progression of the megacolon. Failure of a response within 48 hours, or any deterioration, should prompt surgical intervention. The surgical mortality on these patients is high, but surgery is their only chance if they fail to respond to medical measures. Patients who do respond are treated as outlined for patients with severe disease. Those patients who do recover are at substantial risk of a second bout of megacolon, with a subsequent acute attack of chronic ulcerative colitis (Cello, 1983).

Stricture

In chronic ulcerative colitis, stricture always raises the prospect of carcinoma. Benign stricture does occur and is not uncommon; 10 per cent is an accepted incidence (Huizenga, 1980). These strictures are apparently caused by scarring. They are partially obstructing, but while the chronic ulcerative colitis is active, the fluid colonic contents pass the stricture without causing symptomatology. With remission of the colitis and the production of formed stools, the partial obstruction can become clinically apparent. Colonoscopy aids in ruling out cancer as an etiology. In the elderly patient stricture can often be managed conservatively. Surgery is the definitive therapy.

Carcinoma of the Colon

Chronic ulcerative colitis of ten years' duration or longer predisposes a patient to the development of carcinoma of the colon. These carcinomas are often of multicentric origin, insidious in onset as all carcinoma are and virulent in their course. The risk is greatest for those with total involvement of the colon and much smaller for those with only segmental disease. As a result there is a relatively limited group of patients in whom surveillance for cancer of the colon has a high priority. This can be carried out with repeated colonoscopies at yearly intervals and with a search through multiple biopsies for dysplasia that would precede the development of cancer. This is highly specialized and not without some controversy. These patients are best handled at a specialized cancer treatment center.

Perforation

Most colon perforations in patients with chronic ulcerative colitis are related to toxic megacolon. In an occasional patient without megacolon, an ulcer will extend through the muscularis and result in a perforation. Unfortunately, the steroid therapy which most of these patients are on tends to mask the symptoms and signs of the perforation. Unexpected deterioration in a patient, even without distention of the transverse colon to diagnostic dimensions, should still prompt a search for free air. The noninvasive imaging techniques facilitate the discovery of small walled-off perforations. Management is surgical; mortality rates are alarmingly high.

Hemorrhage

Bleeding in chronic ulcerative colitis is usually in small volumes but is chronic. Anemia is a regular finding. An occasional patient will bleed massively, and chronic ulcerative colitis should be in the differential diagnosis for massive rectal hemorrhage (Edwards & Truelove, 1964). Usually a deep ulcer will have eroded into an artery.

Amyloid

Chronic ulcerative colitis is a chronic inflammatory disease process capable of smoldering for long intervals. As such, it is in the group of diseases that do give rise to secondary amyloid formation.

Thromboembolism

Venous thrombosis is a recognized complication that occurs during first attacks of chronic ulcerative colitis (Edwards & Truelove, 1964). Thrombosis may involve cerebral vessels or may cause pulmonary embolism (Lam, et al., 1975).

ULCERATIVE PROCTITIS

Ulcerative proctitis is considered by many to be a part of chronic ulcerative colitis. It does have a different natural history and warrants separate consideration.

Pathology and Pathologic Physiology

The pathology of ulcerative proctitis resembles that seen in chronic ulcerative colitis in all ways except the extent of disease and the occurrence of complications. The active disease is confined to the rectum and the sigmoid colon; there is no proximal involvement. Quantitatively the disease is mild. When present, ulcerations are few and shallow. The mechanism of the disease is no clearer than it is for chronic ulcerative colitis. If the mechanism is the same, then there is no clear understanding why in these cases it remains confined to the most distal colon. A few of these cases go on to more proximal involvement and clinically become chronic ulcerative colitis. One study (Powell-Tuck, et al., 1977) demonstrated progression in 5 per cent of patients in five years and 12 per cent at ten years. The remaining patients may have only a single attack or may have recurrent attacks three or four times a year. Some infectious processes, particularly *C. jejuni* infection, can have a clinical appearance that closely mimics ulcerative proctitis. It may be that what we now recognize as ulcerative proctitis is a melange of different etiologies, all with the same expression.

Clinical Presentation

Patients usually present with rectal bleeding and change of bowel habit. Some will have diarrhea; others will have constipation. The bleeding is usually mild, and there may be excessive mucus production. As with all processes affecting the rectum, tenesmus is a common complaint. Systemic signs of disease are lacking. There is usually no fever, weight loss, or sign of toxicity. The extraintestinal manifestations described with chronic ulcerative colitis are not present. The age of onset is commonly in the 20 to 40-year old group, but cases in the elderly are not infrequent. Physical findings are lacking except for some tenderness on deep palpation in the left lower quadrant. An occasional patient with a history of many attacks will have anemia, but there is little else in the way of useful laboratory findings.

Diagnosis and Differential Diagnosis

The diagnosis is suspected when sigmoidoscopy shows involvement of the rectum and sometimes of the sigmoid colon, which stops abruptly and above which appears to be normal mucosa. The affected mucosa appears as described for chronic ulcerative colitis, with a granular appearance and a loss of the normal vascular pattern. Ulcers may or may not be present, but the mucosa will be friable and will bleed when touched (Earnest, 1983). The diagnosis is confirmed by the absence of proximal findings on the barium enema or colonoscopy. In addition, the possibility of an infectious cause needs to be addressed with culture (Table 6–5). The laboratory needs to be alerted to employ appropriate media and techniques for *Campylobacter*. The absence of polymorphonuclear cells on the fecal smear would help give an early indication that *Campylobacter* is not involved. Other possible infections include *Yersinia*, *Clostridium difficile* with toxin production, gonorrhea, *Shigella*, *Salmonella*, or ameba.

An occasional patient may suffer factitial proctitis, but without the patient's cooperation, this is extremely difficult to diagnose. Abuse of enemas, suppositories, and some cathartics can also result in a proctitis.

Management

Since this is a localized disease, it does not warrant aggressive therapy. Systemic steroids are not employed. The various preparations of topical steroids in enemas, foams, and suppositories are all effective. Sulfasalazine in daily doses of 2 gm orally is also effective.

CROHN'S DISEASE OF THE COLON AND RECTUM

Crohn's disease is also a chronic recurrent inflammatory disease, but, unlike chronic ulcerative colitis, it can involve the digestive tract at any level from the mouth to the anus. The colon is a frequent site for involvement with Crohn's disease, and it can be the sole site affected. Crohn's disease of the small intestine was discussed in Chapter 3. While Crohn's disease has its greatest impact in the younger patient, there is a late peak of occurrence, and 10 per cent of patients will have their first attack after age 60 (Goligher, et al., 1968; Harper, et al., 1986). There is a substantial geographical variation in the prevalence of the disease, and there is also significant variation among racial and ethnic groups, none of which has proved to be very helpful in understanding the mechanism of the process.

Pathology and Pathologic Physiology

The impact of the inflammation is on the wall of the intestine, although the mucosa can become involved (see Table 6–3). Granulomas in the wall are frequent but not essential findings. Sparing of the rectum is common. Involvement of the colon and other levels of the intestinal tract is not contiguous, and there are skip areas of involvement separated by areas of normal intestine. The ulcers that do occur are cleft-like and reach down into the wall of the intestine. Where these are frequent, they cut the surface of the mucosa into a cobblestone appearance. This pattern of ulceration is less likely to produce pseudopolyp formation. The deeper, mural site of disease leads to scarring and fibrosis, and stricture formation is a frequent accompaniment. Fistula and abscess formation are also features of this pattern of inflammation.

In biopsies and surgical material, the microscopic appearance is that of a productive submucosal inflammation with a substantial lymphoid reaction. Granuloma frequently are seen.

The full range of extraintestinal manifestations as discussed above for chronic ulcerative colitis also occur in Crohn's disease. Some of these, particularly toxic megacolon, are much less frequent in their occurrence. In spite of the sparing of the rectum from involvement in the disease, there is frequent perianal inflammatory disease with abscess and fistula formation.

The mechanism and underlying cause of the disease are unknown.

Crohn's disease shares many features with chronic ulcerative colitis, including the presence of lymphocytes that are cytotoxic for colon epithelial cells. In spite of the shared features, there are many differences, and the two are best treated as separate entities.

Clinical Presentation

The clinical presentation will differ between those patients in whom the colonic involvement with Crohn's disease accompanies involvement in the small intestine and those patients in whom only the colon is involved. In the elderly, involvement of the colon alone is a more common pattern (Harper, et al., 1986). Involvement of the colon and the small intestine is also more common. Statistical analysis shows only significantly less abdominal pain in elderly patients with Crohn's when compared with younger patients. Most other clinical aspects show little clinical difference in occurrence between younger and older patients. Features studied include diarrhea, weight loss, hematochezia, perianal disease, fever, mass, anemia, leucocytosis, extraintestinal disease, and pain.

The impact of Crohn's on the older patient is related to the concurrence of the disease with other unrelated clinical problems; thus, elderly patients as a group will fare somewhat less well than younger patients with similar degrees of involvement (Harper, et al., 1986). Where the colon alone is involved, the clinical onset is somewhat slower. The serious complication—toxic megacolon—is only a feature of the early stages of Crohn's disease, since scarring and fibrosis in the wall of the colon—a feature of chronic involvement—will limit the ability of the colon to distend.

Management

The general guidelines for management of patients with Crohn's disease do not differ from those with chronic ulcerative colitis. The goal is to obtain a remission. The same drugs are employed, with the primary reliance on sulfasalazine and steroids. Elderly patients have a significantly poorer response to steroid treatment when compared with younger patients (Harper, et al., 1986).

Surgery is carried out for somewhat different reasons in Crohn's disease than in chronic ulcerative colitis. The mural disease with scarring produces obstruction, and the deep cleft-shaped ulcers lead to abscess and fistula formation. The pattern of disease is one of smoldering intractability and development of complications that lead to surgery. Several operations along the course of the disease are common. Severe perianal disease is the leading cause of operation in patients with colonic Crohn's disease; megacolon is second in frequency. Fistula, abscess, and obstruction are more common complications of small intestinal disease, although they can complicate colonic presentations (Farmer, et al., 1985).

Surgery generally involves segmental resection, not total colectomy. The progression of disease to affect previously uninvolved intestine after surgery is a frequently observed pattern. Recurrences are slightly more likely if the initial disease involves both the small intestine and the colon than if it is solely colonic involvement. Patients with perianal disease and fistula are more likely to suffer recurrence (Whelan, et al., 1985). In the younger patient, this nibbling away at the intestine, particularly the small intestine, produces extraordinary problems in management of long-term nutrition. Conservatism in proceeding to surgery is the rule. The same sense of conservatism should apply in dealing with the elderly patient. The remaining life span is shorter, but the intervals between recurrences may also be shorter (Whelan, et al., 1985), and elderly patients with an accumulation of other nutritional problems may fare less well with even minimal surgery.

Once a remission is obtained, medications should be tapered and stopped. The use of low doses of sulfasalazine is not effective in the maintenance of remission in Crohn's disease (Summers, et al., 1979).

Complications and Extraintestinal Manifestations

The range of complications and extraintestinal manifestations in Crohn's disease is the same as that seen in chronic ulcerative colitis (see Table 6–4), but the frequency with which they occur is much different. As indicated above, the scarring in the wall and the deep ulcers produce obstruction, abscess, and fistula formation much more commonly in Crohn's disease. Megacolon is a threat only early in the course, prior to the development of enough fibrosis in the wall of the colon to effectively prevent this complication. Perianal disease, which is not common in chronic ulcerative colitis, is a much more regular finding in Crohn's disease. The perianal lesions, which can include fistula, fissure, and abscess, may present clinically long before the clinical presentation of intestinal disease. In some cases even years may elapse (Huizenga, 1980). Perianal disease is not only less common in chronic ulcerative colitis, but it also does not precede the appearance of the colonic disease. Hemorrhage and pseudopolyp formation are much less common in Crohn's disease than in chronic ulcerative colitis.

Skin, mucous membrane, and eye lesions occur readily in patients with Crohn's disease. Arthritis seems somewhat more common in Crohn's patients, although hepatobiliary lesions seem more frequent with chronic ulcerative colitis. While primary sclerosing cholangitis has a particular association with chronic ulcerative colitis, renal disease is more often associated with Crohn's disease. The inflammatory complications in Crohn's disease can extend to produce obstruction of the ureter with hydronephrosis. Renal stones seem related to ileal dysfunction, and thus they would not occur in a Crohn's colitis without small intestinal involvement.

Crohn's disease shares with chronic ulcerative colitis an increase in the risk of development of cancer of the colon. There is also an increased risk of the development of cancers at other sites in the digestive tract (Gyde, et al., 1980). There is some argument concerning whether the risk to Crohn's patients is as high as that for patients with chronic ulcerative colitis, but the risk in any case is significant and imposes an obligation for surveillance of the patient.

ANTIBIOTIC-ASSOCIATED COLITIS

Antibiotic-associated colitis is synonymous with pseudomembranous colitis caused by the toxin of *C. difficile*. Antibiotics can produce a variety of diarrheal syndromes, but these are usually not associated with colitis. A number of drugs other than antibiotics do cause colitis, but this is not a common occurrence (Thayer & Denucci, 1988c).

Pathology and Pathologic Physiology

C. difficile is an uncommon but not rare constituent of normal intestinal flora (Aronsson, et al., 1985; Bartlett, 1979), and it is not identified by the routine cultures. The organism produces several toxins including a cytotoxin. It is not clear what role if any these toxins play in the development of pseudomembranous colitis. Assay for the cytotoxin is used as an alternative to isolation in establishing the diagnosis. In the absence of antibiotics, the organism does not seem to cause disease. In the presence of antibiotics, and these may be administered by any route but most commonly orally, the syndrome of pseudomembranous colitis can result (Trnka & Lamont, 1984).

The colitis usually has its onset during the course of treatment with the antibiotic four to nine days after the drug is started. Shorter incubation periods are described, as are much longer ones (Tedesco, et al., 1974). The colitis may follow the cessation of antibiotic therapy by as much as two to three weeks and will vary in severity and extent. Pseudomembranes do not always form. The gross and microscopic lesion is that of erosion of the mucosa at the site of the pseudomembranes. There is little evidence of inflammation below the level of the mucosa.

Clinical Presentation

The onset is with the typical symptoms of colitis. Most patients have diarrhea with associated cramping abdominal pain. In a few cases there will be blood in the stool. Fever is a common finding. Palpation of the abdomen will reveal tenderness, and on occasion there may be signs of peritoneal irritation.

Laboratory studies will show leucocytosis. If the diarrhea is severe and/or prolonged, there will be evidence of dehydration (Tedesco, et al., 1974). Fecal white cells, predominantly polys, are present (Quinn & Schuffler, 1988).

Diagnosis and Differential Diagnosis

The diagnosis should be suspected in any patient who develops diarrhea during or following antibiotic therapy. The finding of a pseudomembrane at the time of sigmoidoscopy is highly suggestive of the diagnosis that can be confirmed with a biopsy. The flexible sigmoidoscope passed to its full 60 cm length will miss less than 10 per cent of the pseudomembranes in affected patients. With special provisions for culture, C. difficile can be isolated to confirm the diagnosis. Toxin assay, which is sensitive and specific for C. difficile toxin, can also confirm the diagnosis (Quinn & Schuffler, 1988).

Management

The treatment of choice is oral vancomycin. Dosages reported effective have varied from 0.5 to 2 gm daily for one to two weeks. Relapses do occur and warrants a longer, more involved treatment schedule with vancomycin. In patients unable to take vancomycin, several alternatives exist. Simply stopping the antibiotics and allowing spontaneous resolution is effective in mild cases. Alternative antibiotic regimens have been used, but none has been fully tested. Cholestyramine resin will bind the toxin and has been used to treat this colitis. The dose reported was 4 gm of resin orally four times daily (Kreutzer & Milligan, 1978).

RADIATION PROCTOCOLITIS

The entire intestinal tract is susceptible to damage from ionizing radiation. The treatment of both prostatic, uterine, and cervical malignancy has relied heavily on the use of radiation in the past, and the advent of newer modalities of therapy has not eliminated the use of radiation. Radiation damage of the rectum and colon is a problem in the elderly. Tumors increase in frequency with aging, and the success in therapy permits survival well into the period when late intestinal complications of treatment can develop. Intestinal disease secondary to irradiation has two clinically separate presentations, acute and chronic, and these will be considered separately. In fact, these intestinal changes move along a continuum, and one's speed of progression may be controlled by several variables. Radiation dose and technique play a large role in the development of symptoms. Equally important, but much less susceptible to quantification, are the anatomical lie of the intestine in the pelvis and the occurrence of other intercurrent diseases. Since many of the late changes are vascular, this is of great importance in the elderly in whom cardiac disease, arteriosclerosis, and diabetes may add to the vascular compromise.

The anatomical positioning of the rectum and of the sigmoid colon in the pelvis makes them regular participants in postirradiation syndromes. Loops of large and particularly of small intestine are often included in the fields of irradiation, and changes in these more proximal loops account for much of the variability in both symptoms and response observed from patient to patient. Although there have been great advances in the technique of radiation therapy directed toward limiting intestinal damage, it does still occur.

Pathology and Pathologic Physiology

The tissues of the intestinal wall vary in their sensitivity to ionizing radiation (Earnest & Trier, 1983). The epithelial cells of the mucosa and the endothelial cells lining the arterioles are highly susceptible to damage and underlie most of the clinical change seen. While lesser doses have been shown to cause clinical problems, a dose of 5000 rads is required to produce clinically evident damage to the intestine (Novak, et al., 1979). The acute changes are cell death in the mucosal epithelium with resulting proctitis and colitis. Edema, inflammatory cell infiltration, and shortening of the crypts are all described changes. Ulceration will ultimately occur if the course of radiation is long enough. With cessation of radiation, these acute changes will heal by re-epithelization.

Vascular changes occur as a result of the swelling of the endothelial lining cells in arterioles with encroachment on the lumen. This will occur within months to a year after the radiation. The result is a microischemia involving the colonic wall (Ackerman, 1972). The late changes—stricture, fistula, and abscess—are consequences of these vascular changes. The other very late sequela described is the development of cancer in the irradiated segment of the colon.

Clinical Presentation

Acute radiation damage in the rectum and sigmoid colon is manifest by the onset of proctocolitis. Diarrhea and tenesmus are the hallmark symptoms. Inflammatory infiltration in the rectum reduces its tolerable capacity, and frequent stools with small volume are a result. These are accompanied with some increase in mucus production, but gross or occult blood will not be present until later in the course of radiation. There may be cramping discomfort associated with the diarrheal stools (Novak, et al., 1979). If there is substantial proximal damage to the intestine, the symptom pattern may change. With involvement of the small intestine, particularly the distal ileum, there may be an interference in the absorption of bile acids. As conjugated bile acids pass into the colon, they will be deconjugated by resident bacteria, and the resultant deconjugated bile acids serve as a cathartic. Watery diarrhea is the result. There is little to be found on physical examination except for some discomfort in lower quadrants on deep palpation. Proctosigmoidoscopy will show nonspecific changes associated with proctocolitis.

Late changes associated with radiation are either related to vascular compromise or the development of a tumor. The vascular changes can lead to stricture. If the stricture either is tight enough or involves a long enough segment of colon, then partial obstruction will result. Postirradiation stricture, insidious and slow in onset, is always in the differential diagnosis of constipation. An occasional patient will present with chronic megacolon (Palmer & Bush, 1976). Ulceration with or without stenosis may occur and may lead to the development of perforation, fistula formation, and/or abscess formation. The development of cancer in an area of irradiated bowel is not common but has been reported (DeCosse, et al., 1969; Greenwald, et al., 1978).

Diagnosis and Differential Diagnosis

Acute proctocolitis secondary to irradiation is not much of a diagnostic challenge. The proximity in time to the radiation prompts the diagnosis, and, in fact, one needs to take care that other possible causes of proctocolitis or rectal bleeding are not overlooked in the assumption of cause and effect related to the radiation therapy. Usually, diagnostic sigmoidoscopy and a stool culture will suffice to narrow the diagnosis. While rectal bleeding is expected with radiation proctitis, unusually brisk bleeding raises the specter of some other bleeding source.

Chronic changes produce a much greater problem in diagnosis. Careful barium enema and colonoscopy are the two studies that are generally necessary to clarify the diagnosis. In a patient with stricture and partial obstruction, cleansing to permit adequate study will require care and patience. Generally the x-ray will be of most help in evaluation of fistula. The radiological appearance of ulcers and stricture leaves some doubt concerning the etiology. In the elderly patient, in whom the development of cancer is an ever-present possibility, the colonoscope offers the best avenue to diagnosis. Abscess formation may be best identified and followed with CAT scan or by nuclear magnetic resonance (NMR).

Management

The acute problem is limited by the length of the course of irradiation; therefore, the focus is on symptomatic management. Rectal steroid application by enema or foam is the cornerstone of management. This is supplemented with the use of antispasmotics, antidiarrheals, bulking agents, and dietary manipulations, particularly the elimination of milk and milk products, as necessary to make the patient comfortable. Where proximal involvement of the small intestine produces a component of bile acid diarrhea, then cholestyramine (Heusinkveld, et al., 1978) can provide symptomatic relief.

Management of later changes is highly individualized to the patient. Conservative management is favored over surgical intervention, since the intestinal wall changes that have permitted the problem to emerge will also interfere with the healing of the intestine following any surgical intervention. Stool softeners and dilatation may aid the patient with stricture. Newer approaches to the use of antimicrobials, particularly metronidazole, may aid in the management of fistula.

ARTERIOVENOUS MALFORMATIONS (AVM, VASCULAR ECTASIA, ANGIODYSPLASIA, VASCULAR DYSPLASIA)

A variety of vascular lesions occur in the intestinal tract. Best recognized are the hemangiomas, benign vascular tumors in several varieties, and the telangiectases, including those produced by the inherited Osler-Weber-Rendu disease. Added to this list is an acquired variety of arteriovenous malformation that is largely a disease of the elderly patient. These arteriovenous malformations were first described by Margulis and coworkers (1960) and have received increasing attention as the cause of colon hemorrhage. Several terms have been employed in referring to this lesion, and several of these have led to confusion with hemangiomas and telangiectases. Arteriovenous malformations have become embedded in common clinical usage, even though the term vascular ectasia proposed by Boley and coworkers (1977a) seems to be more appropriately descriptive. The other terms, angiodysplasia and vascular dysplasia, are used less often.

Arteriovenous malformations have been described in the intestinal tract from the esophagus to the rectum and in patients as young as 3 years of age, although the majority of the lesions occur in the cecum and right colon and in patients over 50 years old. Younger patients often have lesions above the ileocecal valve, and it has been suggested that this represents a separate syndrome (Meyer, et al., 1981).

Pathology and Pathologic Physiology

Arteriovenous malformations develop as individuals age. It is not clear whether they are a result of vascular aging or a vascular response that simply takes time to develop. To date the most elegant studies of the pathophysiology of this lesion have been performed by Boley and coworkers (1977a; 1979). They show a progression of changes in submucosal and mucosal vasculature in the right colon which culminates in a true arteriovenous malformation. The earliest stage is represented by dilatation of a vein in the submucosa. This (dilatation) progresses to include distention of the mucosal capillaries and venules draining into the dilated vein. This lesion can become extensive and can involve the capillary rings surrounding many crypts. Finally, when the precapillary sphincters become incompetent, arterioles feed directly and without impediment into this dilated venous network. The result is a true arteriovenous malformation.

Only in the latter stages is the lesion readily visible on the mucosal surface. Identification of the earlier stages requires special preparation by the pathologist. On section, the mucosal lesion is that of dilated, thin-walled vessels, often with only a layer of endothelial cells separating lumen of vessel from lumen of colon. Dilatation of the submucosal veins seems to begin at the point of penetration into the muscular layers of the colon (Boley, et al., 1977a).

The development of the lesion has been related to chronic intermittent venous occlusion by the contractions of the muscles of the intestinal wall. These contractions are forceful enough to produce venous occlusion but not arterial occlusion, and thus during the period of venous occlusion, arterial inflow would continue with distention of the capillary and venous systems. Gradually, a progressive vascular ectasia forms (Boley, et al., 1977a). However, several problems remain unsolved. It is not clear whether the contractions of the colon musculature which produce the occlusion are normal motility events or if contractions of extraordinary vigor are required. Should the latter be the case, then this could represent another result of a fiber-deficient diet. The location of the lesions, predominantly in the cecum and right colon, which is the largest-in-diameter segment of the intestine, has been attributed to the higher wall tensions achieved during motility events. As the diameter of the colonic segment increases, Laplace's law requires higher wall tensions to achieve a given increase in intraluminal pressure (Guyton, 1986). Venous occlusion would presumably be more complete in the segments with higher wall tensions. No other supportable explanation for the development of ectasias and their distribution has been forthcoming.

Clinical Presentation

The only clinical presentation of arteriovenous malformations occurs when the lesions bleed. The bleeding may range from mild, occult blood loss to massive hemorrhage (Meyer, et al., 1981). A bleeding diverticulum represents an erosion into a nutrient artery. The bleeding arteriovenous malformation is an arteriole-fed venous lesion. As a general rule, to which there are exceptions, arteriovenous malformations do not bleed as briskly as diverticula. The lower end of the scale is not well explored. Recurrent episodes of occult bleeding in small volume will produce iron deficiency anemia without much in the way of a demonstrable bleeding source on routine studies. Iron deficiency anemia is a common finding in the elderly, and it is not likely that it will ever be clear how much of it should be ascribed to arteriovenous malformations.

Gross rectal bleeding from arteriovenous malformations tends to be painless except for slight cramping associated with the bowel movement. The slow bleed into the large capacity colon may cause the first symptoms to be of hypovolemia, usually postural syncope. With chronic repeated blood loss, the only signs and symptoms are those associated with worsening anemia.

Diagnosis and Differential Diagnosis

There are only two effective tools for visualization of arteriovenous malformations in the clinical setting—angiography and colonic endoscopy. The two techniques are complementary, not exclusive of one another. Barium contrast x-rays cannot visualize these mucosal lesions, and the surgeon, approaching the colon from the serosal surface, has no indication of the location of these mucosal lesions.

The criteria employed for the angiographic diagnosis of arteriovenous malformations are the presence of a slowly emptying vein, the presence of a vascular tuft (seen in the arterial phase and located at the end of a branch of the ileocolic artery), or the presence of an early filling vein (Boley, et al., 1977b; Meyer, et al., 1981). A slowly emptying vein reflects the delay of contrast in the vascular ectasia, resulting in late arrival and late opacification of the draining vein. This is the most frequent finding. A vascular tuft represents visualization of the ectasia itself. An early filling vein indicates the final development of an arteriovenous shunt that permits early entrance of the contrast into the draining vein (Boley, et al., 1977b). All of these findings identify the presence of an arteriovenous malformation, not the presence of a bleeding lesion. This would require the demonstration of the passage of contrast material into the lumen of the colon, a diagnostic finding in diverticular hemorrhage. This is occasionally seen with arteriovenous malformations but is not a regular finding. The arteriographic finding is that of a potentially bleeding lesion.

Endoscopy permits the direct identification of arteriovenous malformations because the view is from the mucosal side. A bleeding or recently bleeding arteriovenous malformation is associated with erosion and evidence of hemorrhage. Arteriovenous malformations are multiple and can be small, 1 to 3 mm in diameter. Even with careful endoscopy, it is difficult to be sure that such small lesions are not missed in the folds of the colon. Endoscopy seems to have its role in the evaluation of the acutely bleeding patient in whom the source of the bleeding can be identified and in some patients who are treated with one of the modes of cautery (Howard, et al., 1981). If the bleeding lesion is not found but arteriovenous malformations are identified, then at least a presumptive bleeding site is diagnosed and other potential sources for bleeding (cancer, polyps, or ulcerations) are eliminated.

The diagnostic pathway for a patient with an acute bleed should provide first for stabilization of the patient's condition with necessary fluid replacement, transfusion, and the like. In addition to a CBC and panel chemistries, blood should be drawn for coagulation studies. Nasogastric aspiration gives some clue to the presence of upper gastrointestinal bleeding. Sigmoidoscopy should rule out the presence of low lying cancer, hemorrhoids, fissure, inflammatory bowel disease, or rectal ulcer as a cause of the bleeding. A plain film of the abdomen should be obtained. At this point if the colon can be cleansed adequately, then colonoscopy is in order. Oral lavage using one of the nonabsorbable lavage solutions can be safely carried out in the elderly. The colon can be prepared for endoscopy in two hours or less (Gostout,

1988). Newer instruments with large capacity suction channels can complete the preparation and permit careful inspection of the mucosa. Should colonoscopy fail to identify a lesion or not be performed for technical reasons, then angiography is the procedure of choice. If, on completion of these studies the diagnosis remains in doubt, barium contrast x-rays may be in order (Brandt & Boley, 1984).

Differentiation of the bleeding from arteriovenous malformations and from other possible diagnoses is relatively clear with the above protocol except in the patient in whom active bleeding has stopped and in whom both diverticula and arteriovenous malformations are present.

Management

Most bleeding arteriovenous malformations stop spontaneously. In the unusual case with continuing hemorrhage, one can take advantage of whatever diagnostic tool has identified the site of the hemorrhage. With a selective angiographic catheter in place, selective infusion of vasoconstrictor agents will arrest the hemorrhage (Brandt, 1984). If the bleeding lesion is discovered at the time of endoscopy, the use of one of the cautery modes is in order. Laser, electrocautery, and the heater probe have all proven effective (Bynum & Jacobson, 1988). If the bleeding site cannot be identified, then one must resort to surgery, most often a hemicolectomy.

The problem often is not with the acute bleed but with the recurrence of bleeds. Frequently there is an assortment of arteriovenous malformations identified with or without accompanying diverticula, but the bleeding site remains unidentified. It is possible to attempt to cauterize likely lesions, but there is little guarantee that this will catch the right site and it is not without some risk. Right hemicolectomy has been advocated in the past, but arteriovenous malformations do occur in both the small intestine and the left colon; therefore, there is no assurance that this will be effective and it too has major risk factors associated with the procedure, particularly in the elderly patient. The management of each patient with recurrent bleeding must be individualized to that patient's circumstances.

TUMORS

Tumors commonly occur in the colon and rectum. Benign tumors may cause some minor blood loss, but most are clinically silent. Adenomas are believed to represent premalignant lesions, clinically silent but not insignificant. Malignant colon tumors are second only to lung cancer as a cause of cancer mortality in the United States. Both benign and malignant tumors of the colon increase in frequency with age, a feature that they share with tumors in general (Lipschitz, et al., 1985). The incidence of tumor, particularly premalignant tumors, is high enough to prompt consideration of screening in high-risk groups. The elderly are included in the high-risk category.

While most clinical attention is directed toward adenomatous polyps and adenocarcinoma, the colon is host to a much larger variety of tumors (Table 6–6). In addition to these tumors, there are rare tumors including anal carcinoma, squamous cell carcinoma, leiomyosarcoma, leiomyomas, and malignant melanoma of the anus. These rare lesions will not be considered further.

In addition to the true neoplasms, there are a number of pseudo-tumors that can occur in the colon and should be entered into the differential diagnosis of colon lesions. These include the polyps in Cronkhite-Canada syndrome, amebomas, tuberculomas, and pseudo-polyps in inflammatory bowel disease.

Adenomatous Polyps

Adenomatous polyps come in several varieties—simple or tubular adenomas, villous adenomas, and a mixed villotubular adenoma. In the United States adenomatous polyps are the most common tumors in the digestive tract. There is great regional variation, and in some areas of the world these tumors are rare. Most of the interest focused on adenomatous polyps is in reference to their potential for malignant change.

Pathology and Pathologic Physiology

These are true tumors arising from the mucosal epithelium. The pattern of growth may produce a sessile polyp or a pedunculated adenoma. Simple adenoma appears as closely packed masses of colonic glands which will show varying degrees of glandular and cellular atypia. Glands may branch, and the orderly maturation of cells may be disturbed. Cellular atypia is often manifest. In villous adenomas the

TABLE 6–6. Tumors of the Colon

Benign	Malignant
Polyps	Adenocarcinoma
Simple adenomas	Annular
Villous adenomas	Polypoid
Mixed	Lymphoma
Hyperplastic	Carcinoid
Lipoma	Squamous cell carcinoma
Hemangioma	

cells are no longer found in tubular gland-like structures but are reoriented into a finger-like villous pattern. In both varieties of tumor, the goblet cells retain their ability to secrete mucus; in the villous adenoma this can achieve clinically significant quantities. Many tumors contain both elements and are called mixed tumors.

The degree of dysplasia varies, and tumors containing villous elements tend to have more evidence of dysplasia. While carcinomatous change can occur in colonic mucosa, in the absence of polyp formation it appears that the largest number of colon carcinomas arise from polyps (Radi & Fenoglio-Preiser, 1988).

The wide geographical variation in the occurrence of adenomatous polyps suggests that the underlying mechanism is an environmental carcinogen ingested with food or water and, with a prolonged exposure to the mucosal cells, initiates tumor growth. The low incidence of the tumor in individuals who subsist on high fiber diets has led to the hypothesis that the slowing of the transit, which occurs as bulk is refined out of the diet, permits prolonged contact of mucosa with an ingested carcinogen. The cause and effect relationship remains speculative.

There are a number of syndromes of multiple polyposis, but only in familial polyposis, Gardner's syndrome, and Turcot's syndrome are the polyps adenomatous. Few of these lesions remain undiscovered in patients past age 50. It is not a disease of the elderly.

Clinical Presentation

Small polyps are clinically silent. Polyps larger than one centimeter may bleed, and as they grow, larger polyps may cause obstruction. Low-lying polyps may prolapse through the anus. Villous adenomas, particularly large ones, may produce prodigious amounts of mucus. If these tumors are low lying (within 20 centimeters of the anus), this can cause mucorrhea with potassium loss sufficient to produce clinical symptoms of hypokalemia.

Diagnosis and Differential Diagnosis

The two approaches to diagnosing polyps are by barium contrast x-ray and by endoscopy. Large polyps are relatively easy to detect with either method. The greatest concern is in the detection of small polyps that have not had enough time to undergo malignant degeneration. Only the air contrast barium enema is sensitive enough for radiological detection of these small polyps. There has been ongoing discussion concerning whether the endoscopic or radiological approach to detection is more sensitive and, thus, preferable. Both methods seem to have a high degree of sensitivity, detecting 90 per cent of the polyps

(Fork, 1981). X-ray studies seem to be somewhat easier to perform and have fewer complications. Colonoscopy offers not only an excellent diagnostic yield but an opportunity to biopsy and/or remove the polyp. The balance at present seems to favor colonoscopy, but when incomplete for whatever reason, air contrast barium enema becomes a necessary complementary study. Once the polyp is identified, biopsy, preferably by excision through a colonoscope, is essential to confirm the diagnosis.

Management

Removal is the preferred management of adenomatous polyps; failing that, they should be biopsied. Patients unable to tolerate colonoscopy for removal or biopsy are frequently also unable to tolerate direct surgical attack on the tumor. Polyps under one centimeter in diameter which cannot be removed through the endoscope because of technical problems in approaching the lesion pose particular problems. It is unlikely to be cancerous but it does retain a potential for malignant change. The decision to proceed to surgery or to institute frequent careful follow-up with air contrast barium enema will be affected by the patient's age and current health, the presence of other intercurrent medical problems, and the size and appearance of the tumor on x-ray. Each case must be individualized. Larger tumors deserve removal. If size or position precludes endoscopic removal, then surgery should be considered. Again factors of age and other medical problems will play a large role in determining the management.

Patients who have been diagnosed as having an adenomatous polyp represent a group of individuals with known instability of the mucosa. They are in fact in a high-risk group for the development of colon carcinoma. One careful review (Lotfi, et al., 1986) placed the risk of the development of carcinoma of the colon in patients who have had at least one polyp at 2.7 times that of the general population. This is a significant risk, and the risk is higher if patients have had several polyps and particularly if more than one segment of the colon is involved. Cancer when it develops may be at some distance from the previously removed polyp.

Lipoma

These submucosal tumors are found in the colon more commonly than elsewhere in the digestive tract. They are solitary lesions and tend to occur more commonly in the right colon. Lipomas of the ileocecal valve are well described. The peak incidence is in the elderly patient (Brandt, 1984). Since these fatty tumors are radiolucent, their radiological appearance often permits their diagnosis. Lipomas are submucosal, are recognizable only as a filling defect, and are not clearly identifiable through the endoscope. They only become a management problem when very large, at which point surgery is the only recourse.

Hyperplastic Polyp

These common lesions of the rectosigmoid are not clearly neoplastic. The lesion occurs as a result of a delay in the migration of colon epithelial cells which produces a polypoid appearance (Kaye, et al., 1973). They do not appear to be premalignant lesions and, when diagnosed, do not place the patient in a high-risk group for the development of cancer.

Adenocarcinoma

Adenocarcinoma of the colon and rectum rises in incidence with age. Few cancers are found before age 40. The risk increases more sharply after age 50 and doubles with each decade after that (Winawer & Sherlock, 1983). The incidence and the mortality associated with these tumors move them to a category of special consideration in the elderly, and screening of early diagnosis is very much a part of management. In addition to age, there are a number of other predisposing conditions that identify high-risk groups. These include the presence of adenomatous polyps, a diagnosis of ulcerative colitis or regional enteritis, the occurrence of inherited polyposis syndromes, including familial polyposis and Peutz-Jeghers syndrome, and the prior occurrence of genital cancer in women. Younger patients in these high-risk groups may be susceptible to developing colon cancer.

Pathology and Pathologic Physiology

Colorectal carcinoma has wide variation in geographical incidence. This has led to the concept that there are specific environmental factors involved in the development of colon carcinoma. As mentioned above, there are also additional genetic, familial, and other host factors that interact in any given individual to permit the development of the cancer.

Cancers are not evenly distributed in the colon and rectum. There are more tumors in the regions of relative fecal stasis. Over 50 per cent of the tumors arise in the rectum and sigmoid; an additional 15 per cent occur in the cecum. Men have more carcinoma of the rectum and women a slightly higher incidence of colon cancers (Winawer & Sherlock, 1983). The pattern of growth of the tumors may be as a polypoid cancer or as an annular cancer. Annular tumors tend to infiltrate and ulcerate. More polypoid tumors are found on the right side of the colon, and annular tumors predominate on the left (Faintuch & Levin, 1988).

When the glandular elements of the tumor retain the ability to secrete mucin, the cancer is termed mucinous, and the prognosis for cure is somewhat poorer. Much attention focuses on the histological appearance of the tumor in an attempt to predict its future behavior and its curability at the time of diagnosis. Tumors with a natural history of slow growth and delayed metastases may reach remarkable size yet remain curable by resection. Other tumors that are small but have a pattern of early metastases may be beyond cure before any hope of discovery because of the lack of symptom production. Most of the classification systems, which are well developed for colon cancer, attempt to describe pathological criteria that are predictive of the natural history of the cancer. The most widely accepted classification is that originated by Dukes (1932) and subjected to a number of subsequent modifications (Faintuch & Levin, 1988). This classification grades the histological appearance, the anatomical extent of the neoplasm in the bowel wall, and the invasion of vessels and spread beyond the wall of the colon.

Special attention must be paid to mucosal lesions that have not penetrated the muscularis mucosae. Many of these very superficial lesions have come to attention because of the widespread use of colonoscopy. Lesions at this stage are referred to as dysplasia and behave in a benign way (Carlsson, et al., 1986). Classification of these dysplastic lesions has been undertaken (Carlsson, et al., 1986), but their clinical significance is still under investigation.

Clinical Presentation

Generally speaking a carcinoma of the colon has two pathways for mischief prior to spread or metastases. These tumors may either bleed or obstruct the lumen. Bleeding need not be massive, and, in fact, early in the development of the tumor, it is likely to be occult. Bleeding to the point of anemia, with secondary symptoms caused by the anemia, is a common story. Gross bleeding is usually associated with ulcerated tumors.

Annular tumors in particular may produce partial or complete obstruction. This is usually clinically evident for left-sided tumors earlier in the course. The semiliquid colon contents in the right colon are capable of passing obstructive lesions far more easily than the semisolid contents in the left colon. The patient will perceive a change in bowel habits with distention and some abdominal discomfort, usually cramping. Low-lying rectal lesions may produce tenesmus and change in caliber of the stool.

In addition to these local symptoms there are some less well understood systemic symptoms and signs. These include malaise, anorexia, weight loss, and fatigue.

Spread of the tumor by local invasion can result in infiltration of the bladder, vagina, or anterior abdominal wall, with or without fistula formation. Such spread may also result in intestinal obstruction. Tumor may be palpable as a mass through the anterior abdominal wall. Because the tumors are often low lying, many are within reach of the finger at the time of rectal examination.

Distant metastases may be responsible for a variety of syndromes, and the clinical presentation will depend on the site involved. Tomography with the newer imaging techniques offers an unprecedented opportunity for screening of the liver and the retroperitoneal structures before surgery.

Diagnosis

If there is any clinical suspicion of the presence of cancer, vigorous search is in order. In addition to clinical symptoms, the presence of gross rectal bleeding or the discovery of occult blood in the stool are sufficient indications in the elderly to warrant investigation. The principal tools are the barium enema x-ray and the colonoscope. As is often the case, an air contrast barium enema is more sensitive to the presence of smaller lesions than the full column study. However, when the cancer has advanced to the point of causing clinical symptoms, the conventional barium enema will show the lesion.

Colonoscopy offers the advantage of visualizing small mucosal lesions and permitting the biopsy of any suspicious lesion. In addition to biopsy, there is the opportunity to use brush cytology and occasionally lavage cytology to access suspicious areas. It is important to remember that not all areas of the colon can be viewed during most colonoscopies, and some exams are incomplete because of kinking, partial obstruction, and poor preparation. In many patients only proctosigmoidoscopy can be performed for a variety of reasons. The flexible sigmoidoscope has a distinct advantage over the rigid instrument (Winnan, et al., 1980). The barium enema x-ray and an endoscopic procedure are complementary and do not replace one another.

Management

There are two aspects to the management of carcinoma of the colon. One is the management of patients with a diagnosed tumor; the other involves the management of those patients who fall into a high-risk group for its development.

If the presence of a tumor has been diagnosed, then the major management decision usually hinges on the presence or absence of metastases. In a few patients acute obstruction or perforation is the presenting problem and demands urgent resolution, but these patients are in the minority. The full range of radiological diagnostic tools—isotope scan, CAT scan, NMR imaging, and laparoscopy—now available offers a host of opportunities to individualize the search for metastases in each patient.

In general, patients with demonstrable metastases fall into a category in which the goal is palliative management. There are a number of aggressive protocols that address the management of hepatic metastases. These usually involve some technique of regional perfusion of the liver with chemotherapeutic agents, but in fact all of these provide only palliation. Patients with metastases may still require surgical intervention for relief of obstruction or less commonly for relief of bleeding. There is promise that some of the endoscopically directed cautery techniques, particularly laser therapy, can bring relief to some of these patients without surgery. Palliative approaches may involve radiation therapy, chemotherapy, or a combination of the two.

Radiation therapy is particularly useful in the treatment of advanced carcinoma of the rectum where bleeding and local symptoms of tenesmus can be controlled. Radiation therapy is often the most effective approach to the management of symptomatic metastases, particularly those in brain and bone. There are a number of protocols for pre- or postoperative radiation. The most notable effect seems to be the prolongation of symptom-free intervals (Gastrointestinal Tumor Study Group, 1984). Chemotherapy has not proven itself to be as effective a tool in the treatment of carcinoma of the colon as it has with other tumors, since colon cancer seems to be relatively resistant to this treatment modality. Most attention has focused on combination chemotherapy and the use of chemotherapy in conjunction with radiation therapy. In selected patients these agents seem to provide increased survival, with enhanced quality of life. In patients without evidence of metastases, the surgical removal of the tumor is the only hope of cure. Primary treatment with radiation or chemotherapy has not been effective.

The management of patients who fall in the high-risk category, to prevent the development of tumors or to provide early diagnosis that will permit removal before spread, is central to the care of the elderly patient. Increasing age is one factor that moves patients into a high-risk group. There is also interest in primary prevention, i.e., changes in diet and lifestyle, that will reduce the impact of environmental factors associated with the development of colon carcinoma. There is little evidence that primary prevention could have any significant impact on the current population of elderly patients.

Most approaches at screening of groups with the regular risk of the development of carcinoma of the colon have not been cost effective. Screening for the presence of occult blood in the stool has been the most common approach. While freestanding programs of screening have not been deemed cost effective, the incorporation of screening as a component of general care in the elderly patient is proper. Annual rectal examination and test for occult blood should be a part of the examination of every patient over the age of 40 years who seeks medical care. Sigmoidoscopy at regular intervals is also in order, but there has been some disagreement concerning the frequency. There is general agreement that annual exams are not rewarding until age 60. Patients who enter a high-risk group at a younger age, such as those with inflammatory bowel disease or with demonstrated adenomas, generally warrant more frequent evaluation with both barium enema and colonoscopy.

Screening by the examination of the blood for tumor markers has not yet been shown to be sensitive enough to be effective. These tests have been used in the follow-up of patients after surgery or other therapy, where they may give early evidence of the recurrence of tumors.

Carcinoid Tumor

Carcinoid tumors may be benign or malignant. These tumors develop from argentaffin cells, which are normal constituents of the glandular epithelium. These cells can function and secrete active substances to cause the carcinoid syndrome. In the colon these tumors are often malignant and will metastasize, but if they occur in the rectum they follow a more benign course (Winawer, 1972).

Most of the colonic carcinoids occur in the cecum. They are mass lesions, which like adenocarcinomas can bleed or cause obstruction. The larger the tumor, the more likely it is that it will metastasize. Carcinoid syndrome is not a common accompaniment. Management is surgical excision.

Rectal carcinoids are associated with aging. These tend to behave as benign tumors and are not frequent causes of carcinoid syndrome. Because they are readily accessible to the endoscope, they are often treated with excision and/or fulguration through the endoscope. Only bulky tumors or the rare malignant tumor will require surgical intervention.

Lymphoma

Primary lymphoma of the colon is an uncommon lesion, but those that do occur tend to appear in the elderly patient. Generalized lymphoma does involve the colon in 10 per cent of the patients. Primary involvement presents much as carcinoma of the colon, and often only biopsy or surgical excision will make the diagnosis clear.

RECTAL PROLAPSE

While rectal prolapse can occur in either sex and at any age, there is one subset of the problem which seems to involve elderly women.

Pathology and Pathologic Physiology

Predisposing features for the development of rectal prolapse include laxity of pelvic musculature and ligaments (often a result of multiple pregnancies), dilatation of the anal sphincter (often associated with the presence of third-degree hemorrhoids), and the occurrence of rectocele or vaginocele (Mackle & Parks, 1986). There is ongoing discussion whether rectal prolapse represents a herniation of the colon or an intussusception. In fact either may occur, and in some patients there may be elements of both mechanisms (Altemeier, et al., 1971).

Clinical Presentation and Diagnosis

The presentation is that of the prolapse itself. In some patients this may occur only at the time of bowel movement, while in others lesser stresses will cause the prolapse. Once the prolapse occurs, it usually requires manual reduction.

Management

There is no substitute for surgery in the correction of the prolapse. The use of stool softeners and added bulk in the diet to reduce straining at stool can be helpful in patients who for other reasons are not surgical candidates. These patients are often incontinent, and repair of the prolapse is essential to the management of the incontinence.

REFERENCES

Ackerman, L. V.: The pathology of radiation effect of normal and neoplastic tissue. Am J Roentgenol Rad Ther Nucl Med 114:447–459, 1972.
Altemeier, W. A., et al.: Nineteen years' experience with one-stage perineal repair of rectal prolapse. Ann Surg 173:993–1006, 1971.
Aronsson, B., et al.: Antimicrobial agents and *Clostridium difficile* in acute enteric disease: Epidemiological data from Sweden, 1980–1982. J Infect Dis 151:476–481, 1985.

Athanasoulis, C. A., et al.: Mesenteric arterial infusions of vasopressin for hemorrhage from colonic diverticulosis. Am J Surg 129:212–216, 1975.

Bartlett, J. G.: Antibiotic-associated pseudomembranous colitis. Rev Infect Dis 1:530–539, 1979.

Behringer, G. E., and Albright, N. L.: Diverticular disease of the colon: A frequent cause of massive rectal bleeding. Am J Surg 125:419–423, 1973.

Boley, S. J., et al.: Lower intestinal bleeding in the elderly. Am J Surg 137:57–64, 1979.

Boley, S. J., et al.: On the nature and etiology of vascular ectasias of the colon: Degenerative lesions of aging. Gastroenterology 72:650–660, 1977a.

Boley, S. J., et al.: The pathophysiologic basis for the angiographic signs of vascular ectasias of the colon. Radiology 125:615–621, 1977b.

Bolt, D. E., and Hughes, L. E.: Diverticulitis: A follow-up of 100 cases. Br Med J 1:1205–1209, 1966.

Brandt, L. J.: Gastrointestinal Disorders of the Elderly. New York, Raven Press, 1984.

Brandt, L. J., and Boley, S. J.: The role of colonoscopy in the diagnosis and management of lower intestinal bleeding. Scand J Gastroenterol 19:61–70, 1984.

Bruusgaard, C.: Volvulus of the sigmoid colon and its treatment. Surgery 22:466–478, 1947.

Bynum, T. E., and Jacobson, E. D.: Vascular disorders of the large bowel. In Kirsner, J. B., and Shorter, R. G. (Eds.): Diseases of the Colon, Rectum, and Anal Canal. Baltimore, Williams & Wilkins, 1988, pp. 537–548.

Carlsson, U., et al.: Is colorectal cancer more frequent in Malmo than in other parts of the country: A validation study of the cancer registry. Lakartidningen 83:598–603, 1986.

Cello, J. P.: Ulcerative colitis. In Sleisenger, M. H., and Fordtran, J. S. (Eds.): Gastrointestinal Disease: Pathophysiology Diagnosis Management. 3rd ed. Philadelphia, W. B. Saunders Company, 1983, pp. 1122–1168.

Dardik, H., et al.: Recurrent diverticulitis in a defunctionalized colonic loop. Am J Surg 108:914–916, 1964.

DeCosse, J. J., et al.: The natural history and management of radiation induced injury of the gastrointestinal tract. Ann Surg 170:369–384, 1969.

Dukes, C. E.: The classification of cancer of the rectum. J Pathol Bacteriol 35:323–332, 1932.

Earnest, D. L.: Other diseases of the colon and rectum. In Sleisenger, M. H., and Fordtran, J. S. (Eds.): Gastrointestinal Disease: Pathophysiology Diagnosis Management. 3rd ed. Philadelphia, W. B. Saunders Company, 1983, pp. 1294–1323.

Earnest, D. L., and Trier, J. S.: Radiation enteritis and colitis. In Sleisenger, M. H., and Fordtran, J. S. (Eds.): Gastrointestinal Disease: Pathophysiology Diagnosis Management. 3rd ed. Philadelphia, W. B. Saunders Company, 1983, pp. 1259–1268.

Edwards, F. C., and Truelove, S. C.: The course and prognosis of ulcerative colitis. Gut 4:299–315, 1963.

Edwards, F. C., and Truelove, S. C.: The course and prognosis of ulcerative colitis. Gut 5:1–22, 1964.

Faintuch, J. S., and Levin, B.: Clinical aspects of malignant tumors of the large intestine and anal canal, including therapy. In Kirsner, J. B., and Shorter, R. G. (Eds.): Diseases of the Colon, Rectum, and Anal Canal. Baltimore, Williams & Wilkins, 1988, pp. 395–417.

Farmer, R. G., et al.: Long-term follow-up of patients with Crohn's disease: Relationship between the clinical pattern and prognosis. Gastroenterology 88:1818–1825, 1985.

Faulk, D. L., et al.: Chronic intestinal pseudoobstruction. Gastroenterology 74:922–931, 1978.

Fork, F.: Double contrast enema and colonoscopy in polyp detection. Gut 22:971–977, 1981.

Gallagher, J., and Welch, J. P.: Giant diverticula of the sigmoid colon. Arch Surg 114:1079–1083, 1979.

Gastrointestinal Tumor Study Group: Adjuvant therapy of colon cancer—Results of a prospectively randomized trial. N Engl J Med 310:737–743, 1984.

Gennaro, A. R., and Rosemond, G. P.: Colonic diverticula and hemorrhage. Dis Colon Rectum 16:409–415, 1973.

Glick, S. N., and Laufer, I.: Radiographic methods in the diagnosis of colorectal disease. *In* Kirsner, J. B., and Shorter, R. G. (Eds.): Diseases of the Colon, Rectum, and Anal Canal. Baltimore, Williams & Wilkins, 1988, pp. 183–224.

Goldberger, L. E., and Bookstein, J. J.: Transcatheter embolization for treatment of diverticular hemorrhage. Radiology 122:613–617, 1977.

Goligher, J. D., et al.: Ulcerative Colitis. Baltimore, Williams & Wilkins, 1968.

Goodman, M. J., and Sparberg, M.: Ulcerative Colitis. New York, John Wiley & Sons, 1978.

Gostout, C. J.: Acute gastrointestinal bleeding—a common problem revisited. Mayo Clin Proceed 63:596–604, 1988.

Greenwald, R., et al.: Cancer of the colon as a late sequel of pelvic irradiation. Am J Gastroenterol 69:196–198, 1978.

Gumbs, M. A., et al.: Volvulus of the transverse colon: Reports of cases and review of the literature. Dis Colon Rectum 26:825–828, 1983.

Guyton, A. C.: Textbook of Medical Physiology. 7th ed. Philadelphia, W. B. Saunders Company, 1986.

Gyde, S. N., et al.: Malignancy in Crohn's disease. Gut 21:1024–1029, 1980.

Harper, P. C., et al.: Crohn's disease in the elderly: A statistical comparison with younger patients matched for sex and duration of disease. Arch Intern Med 146:753–755, 1986.

Henderson, M. A., and Small, W. P.: Vesico-colic fistula complicating diverticular disease. Br J Urol 41:314–319, 1969.

Hendrick, J. W.: Treatment of volvulus of the cecum and right colon. Arch Surg 88:364–373, 1964.

Heusinkveld, R. S., et al.: Control of radiation-induced diarrhea with cholestyramine. Int J Radiat Oncol Biol Phys 4:687–690, 1978.

Hines, J. R., et al.: Recurrence and mortality rates in sigmoid volvulus. Surg Gynecol Obstet 124:567–570, 1967.

Hinshaw, D. B., et al.: Volvulus of the cecum or right colon. Am J Surg 98:175–183, 1959.

Hodgson, J. H.: Transverse taeniomyotomy for diverticular disease. Dis Colon Rectum 16:283–289, 1973.

Howard, O. M., et al.: Angiodysplasia. Lancet 2:1340, 1981.

Howship, J., et al.: Pathology of the aging: Diverticular disease. Clin Gastroenterol 14:829–846, 1985.

Hughes, L. E.: Postmortem survey of diverticular disease of the colon. Part I: Diverticulosis and diverticulitis. Gut 10:336–351, 1969.

Hughes, L. E.: Complications of diverticular disease: Inflammation, obstruction and bleeding. Clin Gastroenterol 4:147–170, 1975.

Huizenga, K. A.: Symptoms, signs, and pathophysiology of bowel complications of ulcerative colitis and Crohn's disease. *In* Kirsner, J. B., and Shorter, R. G. (Eds.): Inflammatory Bowel Disease. 2nd ed. Philadelphia, Lea & Febiger, 1980, pp. 203–216.

Hyland, J. M., and Taylor, I.: Does a high fibre diet prevent the complications of diverticular disease? Br J Surg 67:77–79, 1980.

Kaye, G. I., et al.: Comparative electron microscopic features of normal, hyperplastic and adenomatous human colonic epithelium: Variations in cellular structure relative to the process of epithelial differentiation. Gastroenterology 64:926–945, 1973.

Keith, A.: A demonstration on diverticula of the alimentary tract of congenital or of obscure origin. Br Med J 1:376–380, 1910.

Kern, F., Jr.: Extraintestinal complications. *In* Kirsner, J. B., and Shorter, R. G. (Eds.): Inflammatory Bowel Disease. 2nd ed. Philadelphia, Lea & Febiger, 1980, pp. 217–240.

Kirsner, J. B., and Shorter, R. G.: Idiopathic inflammatory bowel disease of the large bowel and anal canal. Part 1: Clinical features. *In* Kirsner, J. B., and Shorter, R. G. (Eds.): Diseases of the Colon, Rectum, and Anal Canal. Baltimore, Williams & Wilkins, 1988, pp. 261–277.

Kreutzer, E. W., and Milligan, F. D.: Treatment of antibiotic-associated pseudomembranous colitis with cholestyramine resin. Johns Hopkins Med J 143:67–72, 1978.

Lam, A., et al.: Coagulation studies in ulcerative colitis and Crohn's disease. Gastroenterology 68:245–251, 1975.

Lipschitz, D. A., et al.: Cancer in the elderly: Basic science and clinical aspects. Ann Intern Med 102:218–228, 1985.

Lotfi, A.M., et al.: Colorectal polyps and the risk of subsequent carcinoma. Mayo Clin Proceed 61:337–343, 1986.

Mackle, E. J., and Parks, T. G.: The pathogenesis and pathophysiology of rectal prolapse and solitary rectal ulcer syndrome. Clin Gastroenterol 15:985–1002, 1986.

Margulis, A. R., et al.: Operative mesenteric arteriography in the search for the site of bleeding in unexplained gastrointestinal hemorrhage: A preliminiary report. Surgery 48:534–539, 1960.

McGuire, H. H., Jr., and Haynes, B. W., Jr.: Massive hemorrhage from diverticulosis of the colon: Guidelines for therapy based on bleeding patterns observed in fifty cases. Ann Surg 175:847–855, 1972.

Mendeloff, A. I.: The epidemiology of idiopathic inflammatory bowel disease. In Kirsner, J. B., and Shorter, R. G. (Eds.): Inflammatory Bowel Disease. 2nd ed. Philadelphia, Lea & Febiger, 1980, pp. 5–22.

Mendeloff, A. I.: Thoughts on the epidemiology of diverticular disease. Clin Gastroenterol 15:855–877, 1986.

Meyer, C. T., et al.: Arteriovenous malformations of the bowel: An analysis of 22 cases and a review of the literature. Medicine 60:36–48, 1981.

Meyers, M. A., et al.: Pathogenesis of bleeding colonic diverticulosis. Gastroenterology 71:577–583, 1976.

Meyers, M. A., et al.: The angioarchitecture of colonic diverticula. Significance in bleeding diverticulosis. Radiology 108:249–261, 1973.

Morson, B. C.: Pathology of diverticular disease of the colon. Clin Gastroenterol 4:37–52, 1975.

Moss, A. A.: Giant sigmoid diverticulum: Clinical and radiographic features. Am J Dig Dis 20:676–683, 1975.

Muhletaler, C. A., et al.: Pathogenesis of giant colonic diverticula. Gastrointest Radiol 6:217–222, 1981.

Nicholas, G. G., et al.: Diagnosis of diverticulitis of the colon: Role of the barium enema in defining pericolic inflammation. Ann Surg 176:205–209, 1972.

Noer, R. J., et al.: Rectal hemorrhage: Moderate and severe. Ann Surg 155:794–805, 1962.

Novak, J. M., et al.: Effects of radiation on the human gastrointestinal tract. J Clin Gastroenterol 1:9–39, 1979.

O'Mara, C. S., et al.: Cecal volvulus: Analysis of 50 patients with long-term follow-up. Curr Surg 37:132–136, 1980.

Palmer, J. A., and Bush, R. S.: Radiation injuries to the bowel associated with the treatment of carcinoma of the cervix. Surgery 80:458–464, 1976.

Parks, T. G.: Natural history of diverticular disease of the colon. Clin Gastroenterol 4:53–69, 1975.

Parks, T. G., and Connell, A. M.: Motility studies in diverticular disease of the colon. Part I: Basal activity and response to food assessed by open-ended tube and miniature balloon techniques. Gut 10:534–542, 1969.

Parks, T. G., and Connell, A. M.: Outcome in 455 patients admitted for treatment of diverticular disease of the colon. Br J Surg 57:775–778, 1970.

Parks, T. G., et al.: Limitations of radiology in the differentiation of diverticulitis and diverticulosis of the colon. Br Med J 2:136–138, 1970.

Peck, D. A., et al.: Diverticular disease of the right colon. Dis Colon Rectum 11:49–54, 1968.

Perry, P. M., and Morson, B. C.: Right-sided diverticulosis of the colon. Br J Surg 58:902–904, 1971.

Powell-Tuck, J., et al.: The prognosis of idiopathic proctitis. Scand J Gastroenterol 12:727–732, 1977.

Quinn, T. C., and Schuffler, M. D.: The clinical aspects of specific infections of the large bowel and anal canal, including the "gay bowel syndrome." In Kirsner, J. B., and Shorter, R. G. (Eds.): Diseases of the Colon, Rectum, and Anal Canal. Baltimore, Williams & Wilkins, 1988, pp. 439–481.

Quinn, W. C.: Gross hemorrhage from presumed diverticular disease of the colon: Results of treatment in 103 patients. Ann Surg 153:851–860, 1961.

Radi, M. J., and Fenoglio-Preiser, C. M.: Colorectal polyps and polyposis syndromes: Pathological features. *In* Kirsner, J. B., and Shorter, R. G. (Eds.): Diseases of the Colon, Rectum, and Anal Canal. Baltimore, Williams & Wilkins, 1988, pp. 317–341.

Reilly, M.: Sigmoidal myotomy for acute diverticulitis. Dis Colon Rectum 8:42–44, 1965.

Reilly, M.: Sigmoid myotomy. Clin Gastroenterol 4:121–145, 1975.

Ritchie, J.: Similarity of bowel distention characteristics in the irritable colon syndrome in diverticulosis (abstract). Gut 18:A990, 1977.

Rogers, B. H. G., et al.: The epidemiologic and demographic characteristics of inflammatory bowel disease: An analysis of a computerized file of 1400 patients. J Chronic Dis 24:743–773, 1971.

Skarin, A.: Chemotherapeutic agents in geriatric patients. *In* Walshe, T. M. (Ed.): Manual of Clinical Problems in Geriatric Medicine. Boston, Little, Brown and Company, 1985, pp. 81–85.

Small, W. P., and Smith, A. N.: Fistula and conditions associated with diverticular disease of the colon. Clin Gastroenterol 4:171–199, 1975.

Smith, A. N., and Shepherd, J.: The strength of the colon wall in diverticular disease (abstract). Br J Surg 63:666A, 1976.

Smith, B.: Effect of irritant purgatives on the myenteric plexus in man and the mouse. Gut 9:139–143, 1968.

Strodel, W. E., et al.: Therapeutic and diagnostic colonoscopy in nonobstructive colonic dilatation. Ann Surg 197:416–421, 1983.

Summers, R. W., et al.: National cooperative Crohn's disease study: Results of drug treatment. Gastroenterology 77:847–869, 1979.

Tedesco, F. J., et al.: Clindamycin-associated colitis: A prospective study. Ann Intern Med 81:429–433, 1974.

Thayer, W. R., Jr., and Denucci, T.: Miscellaneous diseases of the large bowel and anal canal. Part 2: Colonic volvulus. *In* Kirsner, J. B., and Shorter, R. G. (Eds.): Diseases of the Colon, Rectum, and Anal Canal. Baltimore, Williams & Wilkins, 1988a, pp. 563–565.

Thayer, W. R., Jr., and Denucci, T.: Miscellaneous diseases of the large bowel and anal canal. Part 3: Pseudoobstruction of the colon. *In* Kirsner, J. B., and Shorter, R. G. (Eds.): Diseases of the Colon, Rectum, and Anal Canal. Baltimore, Williams & Wilkins, 1988b, pp. 566–567.

Thayer, W. R., Jr., and Denucci, T.: Miscellaneous diseases of the large bowel and anal canal. Part 20: Drug induced colitis. *In* Kirsner, J. B., and Shorter, R. G. (Eds.): Diseases of the Colon, Rectum, and Anal Canal. Baltimore, Williams & Wilkins, 1988c, pp. 593–594.

Thompson, W. G., and Patel, D. G.: Clinical picture of diverticular disease of the colon. Clin Gastroenterol 15:903–916, 1986.

Todd, I. P.: Some aspects of adult megacolon. Proceed R Soc Med 64:561–565, 1971.

Trnka, Y. M., and Lamont, J. T.: *Clostridium difficile* colitis. Adv Intern Med 29:85–107, 1984.

Weinreich, J., and Andersen, D.: Intraluminal pressure in the sigmoid colon. II. Patients with sigmoid diverticula and related conditions. Scand J Gastroenterol 11:581–586, 1976.

Wertkin, M. G., and Aufses, A. H., Jr.: Management of volvulus of the colon. Dis Colon Rectum 21:40–45, 1978.

Whelan, G., et al.: Recurrence after surgery in Crohn's disease: Relationship to location of disease (clinical pattern) and surgical indication. Gastroenterology 88:1826–1833, 1985.

Whiteway, J., and Morson, B. C.: Elastosis in diverticular disease of the sigmoid colon. Gut 26:258–266, 1985.

Winawer, S. J.: The carcinoid challenge: An interdisciplinary symposium. Memorial Sloan-Kettering Cancer Center Clinical Bulletin 2:123, 1972.

Winawer, S. J., and Sherlock, P.: Malignant neoplasms of the small and large intestine. *In* Sleisenger, M. H., Fordtran, J. S. (Eds.): Gastrointestinal Diseases: Pathophysiology Diagnosis Management. 3rd ed. Philadelphia, W. B. Saunders Company, 1983, pp. 1220–1249.

Winnan, G., et al.: Superiority of the flexible to the rigid sigmoidoscope in routine proctosigmoidoscopy. N Engl J Med 302:1011–1012, 1980.

Winzelberg, G. G., et al.: Radionuclide localization of lower gastrointestinal hemorrhage. Radiology 139:465–469, 1981.

Chapter 7
HEPATOBILIARY DISORDERS

William P. Boyd, Jr.

This discussion of hepatic and biliary disturbance will keep with the theme of this book; that is, it will be limited to those disorders that are of particular concern in evaluating and treating the older patient. Diseases that have no specific relevance to the geriatric patient either are omitted or are discussed with an economy of words. In contradistinction to many other organs, those of the hepatobiliary system do not cause problems for the elderly patient because of diseases that are degenerative in nature, such as functional failure and carcinoma. Rather, the elderly are at heightened risk from disease that also occur in young patients and from secondary, extrahepatic events that stem from senescence in other organ systems.

THE VENERABLE LIVER

From a pragmatic viewpoint there are minimal changes in the liver which occur with aging. There are subtle parenchymal changes, such as an overall decrease in liver weight (despite an increase in individual liver cell size) and an increase of mononuclear cells in the portal area (Shaffner & Popper, 1959). Functional changes are less readily demonstrated than one would expect. It is generally agreed that there is a decrease in hepatic blood flow (Zurcher, et al., 1982). The cause of the reduction is not clear and may be due either to the overall decrease in liver size or to a decrease in cardiac output. Surveys of liver tests (e.g., serum transaminases, serum bilirubin, BSP retention, and so forth)

183

have yielded conflicting results. Suffice it to say that there are no clear significant changes in the standard liver tests due to aging per se.

DRUGS AND THE LIVER

Although one might anticipate important changes in the liver's ability to handle drugs, there are relatively minor changes in drug metabolism due to age. The primary demonstrable effect is a decrease in the liver's ability to oxidize drugs, which affects the drug's serum level and, of course, its half-life. Drugs that are simply conjugated are unaffected in patients of advanced age (Greenblatt, et al., 1979). This is perhaps most significant in the minor tranquilizers. Diazepam is a drug that, because it is metabolized by the mixed function oxidase system, can be demonstrated to have a prolonged half-life; therefore, higher serum levels may result. Lorazepam, on the other hand, requires only conjugation, and consequently steady state is achieved. It is worth noting that a drug's metabolism is not the only consideration in determining its effects. Because the end-organ response to drugs may be altered in the elderly, one cannot use any drug with impunity simply because its metabolism is unaltered. This is particularly true of psychotherapeutic agents, since the sensitivity to these agents is heightened in the elderly.

Certain drugs behave sufficiently distinctly in the elderly patient to merit individual comment. *Isoniazid* is more likely to produce hepatotoxicity in an older individual. The risk of significant hepatic injury is as follows: under age 15, 0.6 percent; 15–34, 2.1 percent; 35–54, 2.8 percent; over 55, 3.5 percent (Dash, et al., 1980). Isoniazid produces a toxic metabolite that is insignificant in most patients; but in a few, the host is unable to detoxify this product and injury results. This appears to represent a most common medical paradigm of a balance between a potential toxin and the host defense. The balance may be upset by producing more toxin by enzyme induction (i.e., rifampin) or by altering the host defense (? age). This mechanism of isoniazid toxicity has been classified as metabolic idiosyncrasy by Zimmerman (1978). The exact reason for an age relationship to hepatotoxicity is not known. Acetylation rates are not affected by age and, in the case of isoniazid, do not explain the difference between those individuals who exhibit significant injury and those who do not.

Other drugs have been noted to exhibit a greater incidence of hepatotoxicity in the elderly.

Dantrolene sodium, an uncommon hepatotoxin, produces a hepatocellular type reaction that is dose- (more common at 300 mg a day) and age- (more common in patients over 30 years old) related (Utili, et al.,

1977). *Halothane hepatitis* also occurs more frequently in the older patient. Certainly the emphasis concerning halothane hepatitis should be placed on understanding the patient at increased risk and avoiding its use in that setting. Patients who have experienced unexplained postoperative fever, jaundice, or especially suggestive transaminase elevation should not receive halothane anesthesia again. Methoxyflurane must also be avoided, since cross reaction may occur. Because halothane hepatitis is much more likely on repeated exposure and is quite rare, it appears likely that the mechanism of injury is hypersensitivity. Against this notion is the inconstant appearance of rash and eosinophilia. Indirect evidence suggests the necessity of an initiating metabolite in anesthetic hepatitis. Halothane undergoes substantial metabolism in the liver and is associated with hepatitis uncommonly; enflurane is metabolized to a lesser extent and produces hepatitis quite rarely; isoflurane undergoes minimal metabolic transformation and does not produce hepatitis (Bradshaw & Ivanetich, 1984). Again we see the role for initial metabolic transformation followed by a host response that causes the injury.

It remains controversial whether steroids are useful in halothane hepatitis. The party line is that they are not helpful; however, data from Varma are rather suggestive (Varma & Kalbfleisch, 1984). The author believes that in situations of significant halothane hepatitis, steroids should be used, since the risk is quite low and we are unlikely to have better data available in the near future.

A recent agent that appears to share an age-related hepatotoxicity is *benoxaprofen*. This drug causes death associated with jaundice and renal failure predominately in the elderly. The hepatic lesion is primarily cholestatic without evidence of severe necrosis or markers of hypersensitivity. This is quite singular in that primarily cholestatic reactions rarely cause death. The most logical explanation of this enigma was reported by Prescott and colleagues (Prescott, et al., 1982). Their hypothesis is that advanced age is associated with a decrease in the drug's metabolism and that the consequent increase in the drug's blood and tissue levels lead to both cholestasis and renal failure. This in turn leads to lethal drug levels causing a toxic death, not one of hepatic failure. In this instance, the liver's role in metabolism may be important in causing the drug injury without the liver itself manifesting the injury (in a lethal sense). This type of complementary role in drug toxicity is most common in drug interactions that lead either to toxicity or ineffectiveness of the agent. Since the elderly take more drugs than younger patients, they are at greater risk for drug interaction.

ACUTE LIVER DISEASE

Acute viral hepatitis in the elderly may be due to all the agents that cause hepatitis in younger patients, but the distribution of the causes is different. Hepatitis A is less common, since in most populations two thirds or more of the elderly have had the infection in the past and are consequently immune. This is easily established by the presence of the convalescent hepatitis A antibody (anti-HAV, IgG). Occasionally one sees hepatitis A in a grandparent who contracted it from a child who is in a school setting.

The lesser incidence of hepatitis B is, on the other hand, more likely due to a decrease in the opportunity to be exposed to the virus. The most common cause of viral hepatitis in the elderly is *non-A, non-B hepatitis*, most often hospital-acquired. A common history is that of transfusion-related hepatitis after surgery.

The assumption has been that viral hepatitis is more often fatal in older patients (Fenster, 1965). More recent data have challenged this concept. Goodson and colleagues reported 23 patients (74 percent of whom had non-A, non-B hepatitis) with acute viral hepatitis without fatality (Goodson, et al., 1982). The treatment of acute viral hepatitis is conservative, supportive care. There is no role for steroids in these patients. Occasionally, a patient will present with a sufficiently cholestatic picture to require biliary tract investigation. We have seen this most commonly in the older patient with non-A, non-B hepatitis. Generally one's suspicion is that the patient has either viral or drug-induced hepatitis, since, despite the marked hyperbilirubinemia, the alkaline phosphatase is not comparably elevated and the transaminases are moderately to significantly elevated. If the laboratory values are indeterminate, a specific evaluation of the biliary tract is indicated. It can usually be accomplished by ultrasound, particularly if the bilirubin is greater than 10 mg per cent (a level at which dilated ducts are virtually uniformly seen if obstruction is present).

In light of the prevalence of extrahepatic disease in the elderly, one must keep in mind that all liver test abnormalities are not due to primary liver disease. Cardiac disease is an important cause of liver enzyme abnormalities, albeit in the main it does not lead to substantial morbidity. Most of the emphasis has been placed on congestive hepatopathy, a well-recognized cause of hepatomegaly and liver enzyme changes. These latter changes generally consist of moderate alkaline phosphatase elevation (two to three times), mild hyperbilirubinemia (1 to 2 mg per cent), and minimal elevation of transaminases (one to three times). Progression of this lesion to significant chronic liver disease is rare, usually occurring in instances of severe prolonged right heart failure (e.g., with constrictive pericarditis or tricuspid insufficiency).

A lesion less well appreciated is that of *ischemic hepatitis* (Bynum, et al., 1979). This lesion has been aptly named from the viewpoint of pathogenesis. The pathologic hallmark of this event is centrilobular necrosis due to the ischemia suffered by those hepatocytes that are at the end of the oxygen line. The clinical presentation is so similar to that of mild viral hepatitis that occasionally a biopsy would be required to make a specific diagnosis. Most commonly, one can diagnose ischemic hepatitis with reasonable confidence simply by observing the clinical setting and evaluating the laboratory results. Generally, these are patients with known heart disease or who have suffered an event associated with hypotension (e.g., myocardial infarction, arrhythmia, and so forth). One caution should be noted: actual hypotension need not be documented in order for this lesion to occur. The laboratory picture is rather consistent. Most patients experience a rapid rise in the transaminases (from several hundred to several thousand) without a concomitant bilirubin elevation. Since bilirubin rises slowly after hepatic injury, it simply does not have time to become elevated by the time of diagnosis. In most situations, the ischemic phase is short lived, the transaminases fall quickly, and the bilirubin does not become significantly elevated. The more difficult clinical situation referred to earlier occurs in patients with poor left ventricular function and presents as a subacute or chronic syndrome that may closely mimic viral hepatitis.

Another relatively common cause of abnormal liver tests from an extrahepatic source is *bacterial infection*, the most notorious of which is lobar pneumonia (Zimmerman, 1979). The laboratory abnormalities reflect cholestasis with mild hyperbilirubinemia and mild elevation of the alkaline phosphatase. This same pattern may be seen in patients with bacteremia of any cause. Histologically there may even be a cholangiolitis. This was first noted by Schottmuler and termed cholangitis lenta; it was believed by him to be the hepatic lesion associated with endocarditis from *Streptococcus viridans* (Schottmuller, 1921). Patients with septic shock have been noted to have not only cholestasis but also this same acute cholangiolitis at autopsy (Banks, et al., 1982; Vyberg & Poulsen, 1984). Several cases and a general discussion of this entity are offered in a paper by Lefkowitch (1987).

Paraneoplastic syndromes do not commonly present as hepatic lesions. The two most common ones are the rare cholestatic reaction in Hodgkin's disease (Levitan, et al, 1961) and in renal cell carcinoma (Stauffer, 1961). In both these situations, there is no tumor in the liver, and the cause of the cholestasis is unknown. In each case the cholestasis disappears with effective therapy.

CHRONIC LIVER DISEASE

Older patients are susceptible to most of the same causes of chronic liver disease as younger patients. A few diseases are unlikely to occur, such as Wilson's disease and primary biliary cirrhosis. The former very rarely presents in older patients; the latter generally occurs in middle-aged patients, although it may persist in rather mild form until older age, at which time it may manifest decompensation.

Alcoholic liver disease in the elderly may initially appear as a more benign process than one usually sees. This is because some patients have modified the amount of alcohol consumed or have quit drinking entirely so that their liver disease is rather well compensated. The presentation then may be that of variceal hemorrhage without prior history of liver disease. These patients appear deceivingly well but in fact may be on the precipice of disaster because of bleeding or hepatic decompensation brought on by bleeding. Certainly one may see the entire spectrum of alcoholic liver disease in the elderly, but I believe the distinguishing factor is the relatively quiescent presentation compared with the more common stormy appearance it makes in the younger patient. One must remember that in this population, alcohol abuse may be a recent problem presenting in a nonhepatic manner. Because of the multiple social problems the elderly may face, closet alcoholism should not be forgotten. The medical difficulties in this situation are those of confusional states, sleeping disorders, and unexplained falls and trauma (Pattee, 1982).

Chronic liver disease from either hepatitis B or non-A, non-B hepatitis plagues the elderly as well as the younger population. As noted previously, the most substantial problem is non-A, non-B hepatitis. It is well recognized that the risk of chronic hepatitis from this virus(es) is higher than the other known agents, affecting two thirds of patients (Sherlock, 1985).

In keeping with the observation that cirrhosis may be quite insidious in the elderly is the observation of "latent" cirrhosis. In a study from the Mayo Clinic, 17 per cent of patients found to have cirrhosis were in this category and 74 per cent of the latent cases were over 60 years of age (Ludwig, et al., 1970). It is unknown whether this represents a special etiological category or is simply a self-fulfilling prophecy representing cases without decompensation who therefore die naturally of nonhepatic causes.

Complications of Chronic Liver Disease

The complications of chronic liver disease are primarily those of portal hypertension such as variceal hemorrhage, ascites, and encephalopathy. One must keep in mind that more subtle complications—muscle wasting, generalized malaise, and easy fatigue—may bring the patient to the physician's attention without overt signs of chronic liver disease. One cannot fail to be impressed by the significant deterioration of general health, at times far exceeding what one would anticipate from the results of the laboratory tests.

Variceal hemorrhage is the most dramatic of the complications and may be the first sign of disease. Endoscopy is always required to make the diagnosis, since all other modalities are less specific. In the evaluation of a significant upper gastrointestinal bleed, endoscopy is the best first test; barium upper gastrointestinal x-ray may be omitted entirely. If the patient is suspected of having liver disease, this is unquestionably the correct course. Another reason that endoscopy should be done is the availability of endoscopic variceal sclerotherapy in the past decade. While shunt surgery is still a viable option for most with noncirrhotic, variceal hemorrhage (splenic vein thrombosis and idiopathic portal hypertension) and for selected patients with good hepatic reserve (Child's A), most patients are best served by endoscopic variceal sclerotherapy. Our experience with this technique in patients over the age of 60 has been quite good, with an overall obliteration rate of more than 80 per cent and a rebleed rate of 10 per cent. The complication rate has been quite low, with the primary problem being esophageal stricture formation (10 per cent), which can be readily managed by dilatation. While mortality studies of sclerotherapy-treated patients are not available in this subpopulation, our knowledge of the natural history of bleeding varices makes it very likely that this approach improves the quality of life if not the quantity. This is not to say that shunt surgery should not be done in this group, but rather that the decision should be carefully considered and even approached with some circumspection. It should be noted that in the acute care of the older patient with variceal bleeding, intravenous Pitressin should be used with care, since cardiovascular complications are common.

The management of ascites in the older patient with cirrhosis is not very different from that in the general population. Because there may be underlying renal insufficiency, one should be cautious with diuretics and, as a general rule, start at lower doses and advance those doses more slowly. Medically recalcitrant ascites is a very difficult problem, and under certain circumstances a peritoneal venous shunt is warranted. Clear benefit from this modality has been demonstrated in some patients, but we have been unable to predict which patients will do well. Generally the best patient is one with otherwise reasonably compensated cirrhosis, excepting recalcitrant ascites and mild renal insufficiency unresponsive to volume expansion. A few generalizations have been commonly observed: acute states of parenchymal failure have a higher complication rate; perioperative mortality averages 10 to 15 per cent; disseminated intravascular coagulation uniformly occurs and may not respond to plasma therapy; and replacement of the valve mechanism because of occlusion is generally necessary every 12 to 18 months. The review by Epstein provides a good overview of this topic (Epstein, 1982).

A major complication of ascites is that of spontaneous bacterial peritonitis. This entity should be considered in any patient with unexplained fever, leucocytosis, or a change in mental status. If either a polymorphonuclear leukocyte count of over 500 cells, a pH of less than 7.35, or an elevated lactate level is noted, then antibiotic therapy should be instituted (Garcia-Tsao, et al., 1985). Even if the ascitic culture subsequently returns negative, therapy should be continued, since culture-negative patients tend to have the same course as culture-positive patients, assuming the original criteria for presumed infection are met (Runyon & Hoefs, 1984). Incidental note is made here of the inadvisability of using aminoglycosides in the cirrhotic patient. The high incidence of renal complications and the present availability of newer antibiotics allow us to avoid this potential problem.

The diagnosis of portal systemic encephalopathy may be more difficult in the elderly than in other populations, since the early symptoms of inattention, disturbance in sleep pattern, and/or mild confusion may be attributed to senility. Consequently, one must remain vigilant to keep hepatic encephalopathy in mind in these patients. It cannot be overemphasized, particularly in patients with known or suspected liver disease, that a good neurological exam should be done to elucidate the cause of any abnormality. One neurological sign—asterixis—is very specific for metabolic encephalopathy as opposed to structural disease (very rare exceptions have been reported). If one finds the aforementioned nonspecific alterations (inattention, sleep disorder, personality change, and so forth) with or without asterixis, then one must pursue this with tests to confirm the hepatic etiology of the disorder. On many occasions one can be rather confident of the diagnosis by the concomitant findings of signs of chronic liver disease and a nonspecific syndrome of encephalopathy without other metabolic derangement (i.e., the exclusion of hypoglycemia, hypoxia, drug effect, and the like). Help may be obtained by the finding of an elevated CSF glutamine level or an abnormal electroencephalogram. The EEG is an underutilized test because it is generally believed to be nonspecific. While this is true as far as sorting out the different causes of metabolic encephalopathy, the EEG is quite good at identifying the presence of encephalopathy and at differentiating metabolic from structural disease. A new way of looking at encephalopathy is by using visual evoked potentials (Zeneroli, et al., 1984). This method of looking at postsynaptic, cellular potential has promise in early diagnosis and patient follow-up.

The treatment of encephalopathy continues to be the combination of removing precipitating causes and of lowering ammonia levels. In the elderly the precipitating cause that deserves emphasis is the use of drugs. Probably more important than the slowed metabolism of various drugs is the enhanced susceptibility to those agents. An erroneous diagnosis of endogenous depression in the patient who is slowed from subtle hepatic encephalopathy will exacerbate the patient's condition if an antidepressant is prescribed. Likewise the use of hypnotics or tranquilizers for a sleep disturbance or the misdiagnosis of dementia will be deleterious for the patient. Other than the avoidance or discontinuation of depressant medications, one must look for the other precipitating causes of encephalopathy such as hemorrhage, electrolyte imbalance, excessive protein intake, constipation, infection, and stress (as from another illness or surgery). The mainstay of the treatment is directed at reducing the ammonia level. The most utilitarian agent is lactulose, which reduces ammonia probably by decreasing its production by bacteria and by increasing its elimination by trapping it in the colon. The goal is to produce two to four loose stools per day. Antibiotics such as neomycin and metronidazole may be used to decrease the bacteria that produce ammonia. Although antibiotics and lactulose would appear logically to be antagonistic, they may act synergistically by acting on different bacterial populations (Weber, et al., 1982). One must be cautious, however, since some patients will be worsened by this combination therapy.

In concert with this approach is the lowering of the intake of protein. In the acute setting the dietary protein is severely restricted to zero to 20 gm per day. This is increased by 10 to 20 gm every two to three days until either tolerance is established or satisfactory protein levels are reached (50 to 60 gm per day). It should be noted that the protein requirement for cirrhotics is the same as for normals. Although controversial, evidence has been found by some investigators that vegetable protein is less likely to produce encephalopathy than animal protein (Uribe, et al., 1982).

The most controversial area in the treatment of encephalopathy is the use of branched chain amino acids. It has been known for some time that there is an alteration in amino acid levels in patients with cirrhosis. In these patients, the aromatic amino acids—tyrosine, phenylalanine and tryptophan—are increased, and the branched chain amino acids—leucine, isoleucine and valine—are decreased (Iob, et al., 1967). There are some experimental data that suggest that this imbalance of amino acids leads to false neurotransmitters and possibly even in an increase in CNS ammonia. In any event, the use of an alimentation solution with a high concentration of branched chain amino acids has been shown to correct the imbalance. Studies designed to evaluate this solution in the treatment of acute encephalopathy in cirrhotic patients have been split as to whether efficacy could be demonstrated (Conn,

1985). In the opinion of most, this solution has not demonstrated clear superiority of standard therapy and, in light of this and its increased expense, should not be used routinely. Parenthetically, it should be noted that many have observed that standard amino acid solutions are better tolerated in the cirrhotic than one would have previously anticipated. The one role for branched chain amino acid therapy appears to be in the rare instance of a patient with chronic encephalopathy who cannot tolerate a minimal protein diet (40 gm) even with the use of lactulose. In this patient, the substitution of an oral supplement of branched chain amino acids will allow a better substantive protein diet without resulting in encephalopathy. This feature of a branched chain amino acid supplement to be less encephalopathogenic than a standard diet has been demonstrated in a controlled trial (Horst, et al., 1984). Although this form of diet is quite expensive, the need for it is quite rare. The vast majority of chronic liver disease patients can be managed by avoiding unnecessary depressant medication, being alert for other precipitating situations, establishing an adequate but not excessive protein diet, and using lactulose judiciously.

In summary, one approaches the complications of chronic liver disease much the same regardless of the patient's age. A few generalizations should be kept in mind. Cirrhosis may be quite insidious in the elderly; therefore, one must be more alert to the possibility that a change in mental status, an anemia or a gastrointestinal bleed, an unexplained infection, or a nonspecific general deterioration may be due to liver disease. Alternatively, just as in a younger patient, it should be remembered that all varices are not due to cirrhosis (e.g., portal or splenic vein thrombosis), all ascites is not hepatic in origin (e.g., peritoneal disease from cancer or tuberculosis), and all confusional states do not signal hepatic encephalopathy (e.g., drug effect).

BILIARY TRACT DISEASE

Gallbladder Disease

Over the past decade there has been a general shift of opinion concerning the advisability of elective cholecystectomy in the asymptomatic patient. Until this time it was accepted that, barring medical contraindication, patients under the age of 60 to 65 should undergo elective surgery for asymptomatic gallstones. This was largely based on anecdotal evidence and studies that were largely comprised of symptomatic patients but that had a small subset of asymptomatic individuals. One oft-quoted study was that of Lund and colleagues, which, while of great interest concerning symptomatic cases, only reported on 34 asymptomatic ones (Lund, 1960). This study reported a 35 per cent incidence of complications over a ten-year period. More recently, several studies have reexamined this issue and have been in general agreement. Typical of these recent reports is the one by Gracie and Ransohoff of 123 persons found to have silent gallstones while undergoing routine health screening at the University of Michigan (Gracie & Ransohoff, 1982). They found the cumulative risk for the development of symptoms to be 10 per cent at five years, 15 per cent at ten years, and 18 per cent at 15 years. No patient died of biliary disease over an 11- to 24-year follow-up. This and other studies indicate that it is reasonable and prudent simply to follow asymptomatic stones. Of the patients who will develop symptoms, most will do so within ten years, generally well before the risk of surgery increases appreciably because of age. The point of this discussion is that if clinicians change their practice habits and decrease the frequency of cholecystectomy in this population, one can anticipate that more elderly patients will have gallstones in the decades to come. This is of some significance because even if the risk of symptoms is low, for those who do develop difficulty, the risk of surgery increases with age.

The overall risk of a cholecystectomy (mortality) is 1.8 per cent based on a survey of 28,000 operations done in Ohio (Arnold, 1970). Glenn reported a 9.8 per cent mortality in the subgroup of patients over 65 years of age in his large personal series (Glenn, 1981). A more optimistic figure was reported by Houghton and colleagues who found in a study of 151 patients over the age of 64 a mortality of 0.77 per cent in elective cases and of 19 per cent in emergency cases (Houghton, et al., 1985). This rather dramatically underscores the significant differences between these subsets of patients in the elderly population. The decision about surgery in the asymptomatic patient will remain a judgmental one, although the weight of the evidence appears to point toward a conservative approach.

Complications of Gallbladder Disease

Cholecystitis in the elderly is little different than in younger patients except that the presentation may be more subtle and the risks greater. In the diagnosis of gallbladder disease, it is most helpful to remember that the symptom is pain. The pain is likely to be midepigastric, as in the right upper quadrant, and occasionally it will be isolated to the midback, the right subscapular area, or the anterior chest. The most helpful quality of the pain is its "restless nature." As opposed to peptic ulcer disease, pancreatitis, and even gut pain, gallbladder pain tends to have a steady but restless nature that prevents the patient from finding a comfortable position. The cramping pain of small bowel disease tends to be more colicky and generally more closely associated with nausea, vomiting, or both. Gallbladder disease may have other elements that are of help, such as a postprandial timing and an associated nausea. Radiation of the pain to the classic subscapular region is helpful when present. As has been repeatedly chronicled, food intolerances (particularly "fatty" foods) have no specificity and are not worth eliciting.

The duration of the discomfort is of some assistance since uncomplicated cholelithiasis should only hurt for several hours, whereas more protracted pain (greater than three hours) implies actual cholecystitis or nongallbladder origin. While generally true, one occasionally sees gallbladder disease with more unusual pain symptoms. It is certainly true that experienced clinicians take little for granted when considering gallbladder disease in the differential of recurrent abdominal pain. The appearance of a cholecystitis is marked by prolonged pain and by the appearance of leucocytosis, fever, or both.

The radiological diagnosis of cholecystitis has undergone some changes in recent years with the advent of uniformly available accurate ultrasonography and hepatobiliary scintigraphy. Just as ultrasonography has become the test of choice in the diagnosis of cholelithiasis in general, it has been quite useful in evaluating the patient with suspected cholecystitis. It is particularly useful in the classic case in which the clinical scenario is so strongly suggestive that all one needs is the confirmation that stones are present. A test that is becoming increasingly effectively utilized is hepatobiliary scintigraphy. This test is essentially a nuclear medicine cholangiogram, since the tracer is excreted by the hepatocytes, affording a reasonable liver scan followed by biliary tract visualization. Since the vast majority of patients with acute cholecystitis have cystic duct obstruction, the straightway appearance of the common bile duct without tracer in the gallbladder defines cystic duct obstruction and therefore cholecystitis with good confidence. The diagnosis of chronic cholecystitis without cystic duct obstruction is more tenuous, but there are indirect signs that may allow the experienced radiologist to suggest this diagnosis. Nevertheless, a diagnosis of chronic cholecystitis by scintiscan should be looked at with circumspection. It should be noted that recent data suggest that scintigraphy may be useful to diagnose common bile duct stones and cholangitis. Again it is noted that the signs are indirect, and the specific diagnosis of common bile duct stones is best made by endoscopic retrograde cholangiography.

Biliary tract lithiasis is appropriately considered as various phenomena along a spectrum, beginning with simple cholelithiasis, followed by acute cholecystitis, then recurrent cholecystitis with choledocholithiasis, followed by the syndromes of lithiasis-related cholangitis. Cholangitis may vary from rather mild cases that abate spontaneously or with antibiotics to severe (suppurative) cases that mandate emergency common duct decompression (endoscopic, percutaneous, or surgical). Cholangitis always means obstruction. At present we consider this obstruction to be stone-related and not to be a symptom of other situations such as biliary stricture, choledochal cyst, and so forth. The diagnosis of a common duct stone begins with clinical suspicion based on the history of pain, fever, and jaundice (Charcot's triad). In more severe cases, lethargy or confusion may be present; this should be considered as a marker of toxicity and should motivate one to immediate action. In less dramatic situations, one may suspect choledocholithiasis from the laboratory studies. Elevation of serum bilirubin may occur without choledocholithiasis, but levels high enough to cause jaundice strongly suggest common duct stone(s). Dumont found that, while patients with mild hyperbilirubinemia (less than 3 mg per cent) had a low incidence of choledocholithiasis (12.5 per cent), patients with bilirubins over 3 mg per cent had a high incidence (69 per cent) (Dumont, 1976). This correlation was strongest in patients with significant hyperbilirubinemia (over 7 mg per cent). The alkaline phosphatase level is frequently elevated in acute cholecystitis and nearly always in cholangitis. Hepatic transaminases are often mildly elevated (less than ten-fold elevation), especially coupled with normal or minimally elevated alkaline phosphatase, suggesting hepatocellular disease and not biliary tract disease. Although an elevated serum amylase level is suggestive of pancreatitis, the elevation may occur in cholecystitis without pancreatitis. Striking elevation of the amylase is quite suggestive of gallstone pancreatitis, particularly if consistent changes in the alkaline phosphatase and bilirubin levels are present.

Surgical Therapy

I will limit my comments about surgical therapy to just a few points germane to the practice of nonsurgeons. As a general rule, most surgeons prefer early surgery in the patient with acute cholecystitis, and certainly surgery within the index hospitalization is preferred over a delay of several months (Lahtinen, et al., 1978). Currently, the area of most intense interest is the evaluation and treatment of choledocholithiasis using endoscopic cholangiography with the potential of sphincterotomy. Certainly in the elderly patient who has had a cholecystectomy and presents with a common bile duct stone, endoscopic sphincterotomy is the treatment of choice (Cotton, 1984). Two issues are possible in the elderly patient with an intact gallbladder and common duct stone(s): either the patient is a good candidate for cholecystectomy or not. If not, then it is reasonable to perform endoscopic sphincterotomy with removal of the stone and to simply follow the patient. In this scenario, experienced endoscopists have achieved good results (i.e., uncomplicated stone extraction, without recurrent cholangitis) in from 75 to 87 per cent (Neoptolemos, et al., 1984; Escourrou, et al., 1984). Late complications occur in approximately 12 per cent (Escourrou, et al., 1984). These results, coupled with the increased risk of common duct exploration, have led some to suggest endoscopic sphincterotomy in patients with common duct stones prior to elective cholecystectomy. This approach will require further study, and these investigations are underway.

Acalculous Cholecystitis

Of particular concern in the elderly patient is acalculous cholecystitis. Since it tends to occur in association with significant other illness, such as sepsis, trauma, metabolic or the postoperative state, the elderly patient is at particular risk. In one series of 68 patients, 80 per cent were over 60 years of age (Fox, et al., 1984). All of these patients had acute upper abdominal pain and tenderness; but it must be emphasized that acalculous cholecystitis is often a difficult diagnosis, and that elderly patients may show minimal signs of the impending disaster. Any right upper quadrant syndrome or even unexplained elevations of liver enzyme tests of appropriate magnitude should raise the suspicion of acalculous cholecystitis. In the report noted above by Fox and colleagues, scintigraphy had a 93 per cent accuracy by revealing failure of gallbladder uptake of the tracer (Fox, et al., 1984). The hepatobiliary scan is not always reliable, however, and the ultrasound can be used as well to look for gallbladder wall thickening usually with distention (Beckman, et al., 1985). In any case, the most important assessment is the clinical one. Taking the clinical setting together with the physical exam and laboratory assessment will allow the experienced clinician to make the diagnosis.

Gallstone Ileus

This is a distinctly uncommon syndrome, but one that deserves mention in light of the relative frequency of bowel obstruction in the elderly. Most patients present with abdominal pain; the presentation is generally after advanced disease has occurred. The diagnosis is often made at surgery, and the prognosis is quite poor.

Cholangiocarcinoma

Although an early diagnosis of carcinoma of the extrahepatic bile ducts is worthwhile because of the slow growth of some of these tumors, the late occurrence of symptoms or signs makes the average prognosis quite poor. The two situations in which signs of disease allow the physician to make an early diagnosis are when obstruction occurs early (primarily in periampullary carcinoma) and when an isolated elevation of the alkaline phosphatase leads to the diagnosis. The most important caveat is that a work-up is indicated if the patient has an unexplained significant elevation of the alkaline phosphatase of hepatic origin. The key word is significant. In the author's opinion, this would be a recent elevation of alkaline phosphatase of more than two-fold proportion. While this is admittedly arbitrary, one must have some pragmatic criterion in order to avoid investigating patients unnecessarily. A prime difficulty here is that the test of choice is the cholangiogram (endoscopic or percutaneous). Anything less is too insensitive to diagnose early cholangiocarcinoma. Whether one agrees with this approach or not, bile duct carcinoma should at least be considered in the differential diagnosis for an elevated alkaline phosphatase in the older patient. One should be cognizant of the myriad of other causes of such an elevation in order to decide if a cholangiogram should be done.

REFERENCES

Arnold, D. J.: 28,621 Cholecystectomies in Ohio: Results of a survey in Ohio hospitals by the gallbladder survey committee, Ohio chapter American College of Surgeons. Am J Surg 119:714–719, 1970.
Banks, J. G., et al.: Liver function in septic shock. J Clin Pathol 35:1249–1252, 1982.
Beckman, I., et al.: Ultrasonographic findings in acute acalculous cholecystitis. Gastrointest Radiol 10:387–389, 1985.
Bradshaw, J. J., and Ivanetich, K. M.: Isoflurane: A comparison of its metabolism by human and rat hepatic cytochrome P-450. Anesth Analg 63:805–813, 1984.
Bynum, TE., et al.: Ischemic hepatitis. Dig Dis Sci 24:129–135, 1979.
Conn, H. O.: Complications of portal hypertension. In Gitnick, G. (Ed.): Current Hepatology. Chicago, Yearbook Medical Publishers, 1985, pp. 391–397.
Cotton, P. B.: Endoscopic management of bile duct stones (apples and oranges). Gut 25:587–597, 1984.
Dash, L. A., et al.: Isoniazid preventive therapy. Am Rev Resp Dis 121:1039–1044, 1980.
Dumont, A. E.: Significance of hyperbilirubinemia in acute cholecystitis. Surg Gynecol Obstet 142:855–857, 1976.
Epstein, M.: Peritoneovenous shunt in the management of ascites and the hepatorenal syndrome. Gastroenterology 82:790–799, 1982.
Escourrou, J., et al.: Early and late complications after endoscopic sphincterotomy for biliary lithiasis with and without the gallbladder "in situ." Gut 25:598–602, 1984.
Fenster, L. F.: Viral hepatitis in the elderly. Gastroenterology 49:262–271, 1965.
Fox, M. S., et al.: Acute acalculous cholecystitis. Surg Gynecol Obstet 159:13–15, 1984.
Garcia-Tsao, G., et al.: The diagnosis of bacterial peritonitis: Comparison of pH, lactate concentration and leukocyte count. Hepatology 5:91–96, 1985.
Glenn, F.: Surgical management of acute cholecystitis in patients 65 years of age and older. Ann Surg 193:56–59, 1981.
Goodson, J. D., et al.: The clinical course of acute hepatitis in the elderly patient. Arch Intern Med 142:1485–1488, 1982.

Gracie, W. A., and Ransohoff, D. F.: The natural history of silent gallstones. New Engl J Med 397:798–800, 1982.

Greenblatt, D. J., et al.: Lorazepam kinetics in the elderly. Clin Pharmacol Ther 26:103–113, 1979.

Horst, D., et al.: Comparison of dietary protein with an oral branched chain-enriched amino acid supplement in chronic portal-systemic encephalopathy: A randomized trial. Hepatology 4:279–287, 1984.

Houghton, P. W. J., et al.: Cholecystectomy in the elderly: A prospective study. Br J Surg 72:220–222, 1985.

Iob, V., et al.: Free amino acids in liver, plasma and muscle of patients with cirrhosis of the liver. J Surg Res 7:41–43, 1967.

Lahtinen, J., et al.: Acute cholecystitis treated by early and delayed surgery: A controlled clinical trial. Scand J Gastroenterol 13:673–678, 1978.

Lefkowitch, J. H.: Bile ductular cholestasis: An ominous histopathologic sign related to sepsis and cholangitis lenta. Human Pathol 13:19–24, 1978.

Levitan, R., et al.: Jaundice in Hodgkin's disease. Am J Med 30:99–111, 1961.

Ludwig, J., et al.: Latent hepatic cirrhosis. Am J Dig Dis 15:7–14, 1970.

Lund, J.: Surgical indications in cholelithiasis: Prophylactic cholecystectomy elucidated on the basis of long-term follow-up on 526 nonoperated cases. Ann Surg 151:153–162, 1960.

Neoptolemos, J. P., et al.: The management of common bile duct calculi by endoscopic sphincterotomy in patients with gallbladders in situ. Br J Surg 71:69–71, 1984.

Pattee, J. J.: Uncovering the elderly "hidden alcoholic." Geriatrics 37:145–146, 1982.

Polk, H. C., Jr.: Carcinoma and the calcified gallbladder. Gastroenterology 50:582–585, 1966.

Prescott, L. P., et al.: Side effects of benoxaprofen. Br Med J 284:1783, 1982.

Runyon, B. A., and Hoefs, J. C.: A culture-negative neutrocytic ascites: A variant of spontaneous bacterial peritonitis. Hepatology 4:1209–1211, 1984.

Safaie-Shirazi, S., and Printen, K. J.: Gallstone ileus: Review of forty cases. J Am Geriatr Soc 20:335–339, 1972.

Schaffner, F., and Popper, H.: Nonspecific reactive hepatitis in aged and infirm people. Am J Dig Dis 4:389–399, 1959.

Schottmuller, T.: Uber cholangitis Munch Med Wehnschr 51:1667, 1921.

Sherlock D: Virus hepatitis. In Diseases of the Liver and Biliary System. Oxford, Blackwell Scientific, 1985, p. 271.

Stauffer, M. H.: Nephrogenic hepatosplenomegaly. Gastroenterology 40:694, 1961.

Uribe, M., et al.: Treatment of chronic portal-systemic encephalopathy with vegetable and animal protein diets: A controlled crossover study. Dig Dis Sci 27:1109–1116, 1982.

Utili, R., et al.: Dantrolene associated hepatic injury. Gastroenterology 72:610–616, 1977.

Varma, R. R., and Kalbfleisch, J. H.: Beneficial effects of corticosteroid therapy in halothane hepatitis: Results of a prospective controlled study. Gastroenterology 86:1345, 1984.

Vyberg, M., and Poulsen, J.: Abnormal bile duct epithelium accompanying septicaemia. Virchows Arch A 402:451–458, 1984.

Weber, F. L., Fr., et al.: Effects of lactulose and neomycin on urea metabolism in cirrhotic subjects. Gastroenterology 82:213–217, 1982.

Zeneroli, M. L., et al.: Visual evoked potential: A diagnostic tool for the assessment of hepatic encephalopathy. Gut 25:291–299, 1984.

Zimmerman, H. J.: Classification of hepatotoxins and mechanisms of toxicity. In Hepatotoxicity. New York, Appleton-Century-Crofts, 1978, p. 93.

Zimmerman, H. J. (Moderator): Jaundice due to bacterial infection. Gastroenterology 77:362–374, 1979.

Zurcher, C., et al.: Possible influence of multiple pathological changes in aging rats on studies of organ aging with emphasis on the liver. In Kitani, K. (Ed.) Liver and Aging. Amsterdam, Elsevier Biomedical, 1982, pp. 19–37.

Index

Note: Page numbers in italic type refer to illustrations; page numbers followed by the letter t refer to tables.

199

Weight loss, adenocarcinoma and, 174
  chronic ulcerative colitis and, 145
  Crohn's disease and, 158
  gluten-sensitive enteropathy and, 52
  peptic ulcer and, 39
  small intestine vascular disease and, 72
  ulcerative proctitis and, 156
White blood cell count, 115, 136
Wilson's disease, 187–188

X-rays. See also *Barium contrast x-ray.*
  chronic ulcerative colitis and, 151

X-rays *(Continued)*
  diverticulitis diagnosis and, 124
  gluten-sensitive enteropathy and, 52
  laxative abuse and, 107
  LES reflux and, 14–15
  rectal contraction and, 102

Yersinia, 156

Zenker's diverticulum, 4